'This well-written book, based on careful a[nalysis of] the current literature on how we think about [domestic abuse on] children and young people, and the longer te[rm impact on the] lifecourse. The book goes beyond the victim/survivor binary, to explore [how] young women have made sense of their childhood experiences, and how their identities have been shaped and reshaped by these experiences. The book is a compelling read. I strongly recommend anyone interested in children and young people's experiences of domestic abuse to read this book – which should be everyone'.

Dr John Devaney, *Professor of Social Work, University of Edinburgh, UK*

'This book is a courageous trailblazer for gender-specific understandings of childhood domestic abuse, focusing on girls' experiences which are often overlooked and silent(ced). Actively leaning into the complexities and tensions of young women's perspectives and rooted in epistemic justice, Dr Frances explores girls' inner worlds. The use of poetry to examine the narratives is enchanting. Written with sensitivity, respect, and reflexivity, Dr Frances holds the narratives like butterflies in her hands. A beautifully written book which offers a beacon of hope for girls to step out of the shadows; they deserve to be heard'.

Dr Jade Levell, *Senior Lecturer in Criminology and Gender Violence, University of Bristol, UK*

'This is a compelling book that critically considers human violence. Tanya Frances has developed a richly narrated critique of domestic violence theory and conveys the power of redressing epistemic injustices where people's lived experiences fall into knowledge gaps. Her research with people who have experienced violence and focus upon its effects is rigorous and holds central, the contributors' experiences. There is precision and power in the presentation of this important textbook and I highly recommend it for people wanting to understand more about domestic abuse or those working within the counselling and mental health professions'.

Lynne Gabriel, *OBE, PhD, Professor of Counselling and Mental Health, York St John University, UK*

NARRATIVES OF CHILDHOOD DOMESTIC VIOLENCE

Narratives of Childhood Domestic Violence explores young women's accounts of transitions to young adulthood after domestic violence in childhood, from a psychological perspective.

This book centres a dialogue about epistemic justice and how experiences of violence that are marginal, marginalised and less easily understood through dominant discourses can be listened to and heard. Taking a critical feminist psychological approach, Frances examines gendered and socio-culturally located narrative practices, arguing that narratives about change and transition in young adulthood after childhood domestic violence both re-inscribe societal narratives that can be constraining and present stories of resistance and hope. This book draws attention to the difficulties of being heard and understood when articulating an experience that sits in tension with normative expectations and trajectories for families and children growing up within them. It also examines how tensions in storytelling practices are articulated in creative, nuanced and diverse ways. Frances ends this book by offering considerations for theory, research and practice, including practical implications and interventions and recommendations for policy.

This is an essential resource for academics and students interested in violence against women, feminist psychology, childhood abuse and concerns around epistemic justice, as well as professionals in counselling, social work, charity work, law and policy making.

Tanya Frances is a lecturer in psychology and counselling at The Open University, UK. She is also a counsellor and psychotherapist in practice. Her research interests and expertise centre around trauma, social inequalities, gender-based violence and domestic violence and abuse. She is a founding member of the Intersectional Violences Research Group, an international group of academics interested in addressing issues around gender-based violence from a feminist psychological perspective.

WOMEN AND PSYCHOLOGY

Series Editor: Jane Ussher

Professor of Women's Health Psychology, University of Western Sydney

This series brings together current theory and research on women and psychology. Drawing on scholarship from a number of different areas of psychology, it bridges the gap between abstract research and the reality of women's lives by integrating theory and practice, research and policy.

Each book addresses a 'cutting edge' issue of research, covering topics such as postnatal depression and eating disorders, and addressing a wide range of theories and methodologies.

The series provides accessible and concise accounts of key issues in the study of women and psychology, and clearly demonstrates the centrality of psychology debates within women's studies or feminism.

Other titles in this series:

Reframing Trauma Through Social Justice
Resisting the Politics of Mainstream Trauma Discourse
Catrina Brown

Narratives of Childhood Domestic Violence
Epistemic Justice, Young Women and Transitions to Young Adulthood
Tanya Frances

For more information about this series, please visit: https://www.routledge.com/Women-and-Psychology/book-series/SE0263

NARRATIVES OF CHILDHOOD DOMESTIC VIOLENCE

Epistemic Justice, Young Women and Transitions to Young Adulthood

Tanya Frances

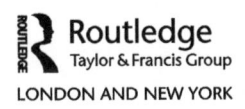

Routledge
Taylor & Francis Group
LONDON AND NEW YORK

Designed cover image: *Assemblage of Life* by Tanya Frances

First published 2025
by Routledge
4 Park Square, Milton Park, Abingdon, Oxon OX14 4RN

and by Routledge
605 Third Avenue, New York, NY 10158

Routledge is an imprint of the Taylor & Francis Group, an informa business

© 2025 Tanya Frances

The right of Tanya Frances to be identified as author of this work has been asserted in accordance with sections 77 and 78 of the Copyright, Designs and Patents Act 1988.

All rights reserved. No part of this book may be reprinted or reproduced or utilised in any form or by any electronic, mechanical, or other means, now known or hereafter invented, including photocopying and recording, or in any information storage or retrieval system, without permission in writing from the publishers.

Trademark notice: Product or corporate names may be trademarks or registered trademarks, and are used only for identification and explanation without intent to infringe.

British Library Cataloguing-in-Publication Data
A catalogue record for this book is available from the British Library

ISBN: 978-1-032-49318-3 (hbk)
ISBN: 978-1-032-49316-9 (pbk)
ISBN: 978-1-003-39316-0 (ebk)

DOI: 10.4324/9781003393160

Typeset in Sabon
by codeMantra

CONTENTS

Acknowledgements ix
Foreword xi
Preface xiii

1 The beginning 1

2 Domestic violence in children's lives 10

3 A feminist psychological perspective on memory, gender and voice/s 28

4 Interviewing women and working with poems 41

5 Transitions 61

6 Recoveries 80

7 Precarious work and creative assemblages of voice/s 100

8 Toward epistemic justice: embodied and reflexive listening 122

9 Staying with and looking ahead 137

Index 149

ACKNOWLEDGEMENTS

To the women I interviewed for this research, I am grateful for your openness and willingness to share your stories.

To communities who have provided spaces for thinking, being and staying with what is difficult when we make sense of violence and its impact. This is not easy work. I especially thank my friends and colleagues, Emma Turley, Lisa Lazard, Lucy Thompson and Lois Donnelly, who are members of the Intersectional Violences Research Group with me, for being part of a working group that holds space for these difficulties and for hope.

I offer this book with hope for continued work that matters.

> Where there is hope, there is difficulty… Hope is not at the expense of struggle but animates a struggle; hope gives us a sense that there is a point to working things out, working things through. Hope does not always point toward the future, but carries us through when the terrain is difficult, when the path we follow makes it harder to proceed. Hope is behind us when we have to work for something to be possible
>
> *(Ahmed, 2017, p. 2)*

FOREWORD

Lisa Lazard

When children living in circumstances of domestic abuse are discussed, they are habitually described as *witnesses* of violence, most commonly perpetrated by fathers against mothers. This timely and much-needed book begins by addressing how this taken-for-granted description of children who encounter violence in their homes is wanting. It does so by reframing the focus from *witnessing* to childhood domestic abuse to experiencing it. This seemingly small shift in perspective is a powerful one that enables the complexities of narrating these experiences – to speak and be heard – to be articulated.

Tanya Frances is one of the few psychologists who meaningfully and explicitly considers the narration of experience of childhood domestic abuse in the context of epistemic justice. Tanya's consideration of this issue is grounded in the complex landscapes of gendered power that mediate and shape what is said, heard and silenced. It comes as no surprise to me that Tanya takes seriously issues of voicing and speaking rights within these frames. I have had the pleasure of working with Tanya on the Psychology of Women and Equalities Committee (British Psychological Society), where we were asked to provide expert consultation on the *Violence Against Women and Girls UK Government Strategy*. Alongside Lois Donnelly, Lucy Thompson, Emma Turley and myself, Tanya established a working group that grappled with questions around victim/survivor speaking rights, the politics of representation and of working in this field ethically and reflexively. As part of this work, Tanya co-founded the Intersectional Violences Research Group in which she has considered questions about victimisation that are attuned to questions of power, ethics and justice when working with victims of gender-based violence more broadly and domestic abuse in particular.

In keeping with a focus on epistemic justice, ethics and power, this book provides an incisive analysis of how we can approach the task of listening to women's stories of their own experiences of childhood domestic abuse. Using a feminist dialogical approach, as well as feminist insights on how we can approach the task of listening, Tanya draws attention to how women's stories of their experiences of childhood domestic abuse are shaped by dominant ways of understanding both children and domestic violence in our current socio-cultural contexts but also how they creatively and meaningfully navigate tensions between dominant understandings of how they should experience their childhood and their own narration of it. This book makes visible the difficulties in articulating experiences that are marginal, less easily understood within dominant sense-making and thus risk being unheard. In doing so, this book captures how children are deeply connected – relationally and affectively – to that violence in ways that go beyond their typical description as witnesses of domestic violence.

This book offers a novel and incredibly important contribution to the field of domestic violence by drawing attentions to the difficulties of being heard and, crucially, comprehended when articulating an experience that sits in tension with normative expectations and trajectories for families and children growing up within them. It is a vital resource for those working with victim/survivors by inviting consideration of survival and recovery that are meaningful for those who have experienced childhood domestic abuse and are framed within concerns about epistemic justice.

PREFACE

When I think about how I arrived at writing this book, the well-known feminist phrase, 'the personal is political' feels like it resonates. As bell hooks articulated, we often come to theory when we want to comprehend our personal struggles (hooks, 1994). This is, in part, the case for me. When I was first working on domestic violence research a bit more than ten years ago now, I worked on a couple of research projects where I interviewed women and children about their experiences of domestic violence. I was also on a clinical placement as a trainee counsellor and psychotherapist at a women's counselling centre and I was volunteering at a domestic violence refuge. I listened to people's stories and tried to help them to understand and make sense of them. I realised one of the things that motivated me to continue this work was my response to listening to women's and children's stories. I was mostly struck by *how* people told their stories. This is not to say that I expected they could not, but I learnt that some of their stories mirrored much of my own. I got curious and started asking myself why I had remained so silent about parts of my own experiences.

I was deeply aware of my own gendered self as a child. I loved medical dramas on TV, particularly the BBC programme Casualty. Perhaps part of me was inspired by watching the show, or perhaps my interest in it came from somewhere else, but I do know that my fantasy was that I would become a medical doctor when I was older. I wanted to learn about people's stories and understand how they had arrived in crisis. I have a particular memory of playing 'doctors and nurses' and coming out with the words: 'I can't possibly play the doctor; I've got ginger hair and freckles, and I am a girl'. Somewhere along the way, I was very aware that my femininity and appearance meant I could not be a doctor, not even in a child's play. I was also labelled a 'shy' child. I understand this now as not shyness but a preference for quietness and peace. Perhaps this is unsurprising in the context of my home life, which was *not* quiet and peaceful. I grew to feel safe in taking up as little space as possible and in aspects of my home life remaining unseen. In some ways, I reflect on my childhood by wondering how I *did* voice my experiences, if my voice was heard when I did express parts of myself, and how parts of my desires and voice became somewhat existing on the margins along the way.

In the context of my own experiences of growing up with domestic violence, I didn't know what sense to make of what was happening, but I did know that it wasn't good. Part of me wanted others to know, and simultaneously, I felt so much shame that I would go to lengths to make myself silent and small so that others would not see. This desire for both visibility and invisibility is striking to me. My own life story isn't the focus of this book, but it does feel important to acknowledge some of where my interest in voice, epistemic practices and childhood experiences of violence comes from.

My experience of childhood, I feel, is captured by that of many other children who grew up with domestic violence and have been described as 'hidden in plain sight'. It has taken me a while to grapple with this. To grapple with my own history and the complicated ways that living with a story that was largely untold, unheard and unrecognised has shaped me in embodied, relational and biographical ways. In my experience, when one's reality is unaccounted for and unrecognised, it can have a big impact on one's sense of the validity of one's own knowledge and the credibility of oneself as a legitimate knower. I should also say that I count myself as fortunate in many ways due to how socio-structural power has afforded me privileges. By this, I mean that I am a white, cis-gender woman with a good education and resources that meet my needs. I am OK. At the same time, I am interested in how we find ways of communicating these stories of both struggle and survival.

I write this book primarily as an academic feminist psychologist. This book is based on interviews I conducted with young adult women living in England who grew up with domestic violence in childhood. It takes a particular interest in voice. I examine the kinds of narrative practices and resources that shape how women voice experiences of violence in childhood and how these stories come to be heard. This research was part of my doctoral research project. However, my thinking is also shaped by my broader understanding of trauma, violence and abuse as an academic, as a clinical practitioner in counselling and psychotherapy and as a person with personal lived experience.

This book draws on feminist psychology and a dialogical way of viewing selfhood and identity to explore how the women I interviewed narrated the self and constructed a sense of self through their stories of living through and living after violence in childhood. This book is about domestic violence, but it is also about voice and how we think about what kind of knowledge counts and from whom. In orienting this book to narrative psychology, I am particularly interested in asking questions about what stories *do*. As such, this book is about what shapes the stories we tell about who we are. It is also about how the stories we tell about who we are can have huge power in shaping what is known about us and how we see ourselves. To stay with these lines of enquiry, recognising that the psychological is political, this book examines the individual life stories of the women I interviewed, as well as the socio-cultural contexts in which experiences of childhood violence are voiced and heard.

Reference

hooks, b. (1994). *Teaching to transgress: Education as the practice of freedom.* Routledge.

1
THE BEGINNING

Introduction

Due to women's and feminist activism, Violence Against Women and Girls (VAWG) is now much more spoken about and named in Global North and Western contexts, in public discourse, and in national and international agendas and legislation that recognise the extent of the problem and aim to tackle it. We are at a time of living through social and cultural movements such as #MeToo (Lazard, 2020; Maier, 2023), with more women coming forward and talking publicly about experiences of men's violence against women. It feels like not a week goes by when the UK media does not publish a news story about misogynistic acts of men's brutal VAWG. Just this week, my news apps alerted me to the arrest of a 17-year-old male on suspicion of murder and attempted murder after a knife attack at a Taylor Swift dance class in Southport, UK. The knife attack resulted in the death of three girls, Bebe King, Elsie Dot Stancombe and Alice Dasilva Aguiar, and injuries to eight other girls and two women dance and yoga teachers. This is one example, but the extent of men's violence against women in the UK context is enormous and costs women and other marginalised people their lives and sense of safety. *The Guardian* launched this year (2024) a 'Killed Women Count' (Topping et al., 2024), which aims to report on every woman killed by a man in the UK, recognising that while some cases do make the news, the majority do not and, therefore, go largely unheard. New names are added to the count on a regular basis.

The National Police Chief's Council (NPCC) released a VAWG National Policing Statement (National Police Chief's Council, 2024), which noted that VAWG has reached an epidemic level in England and Wales, estimating that around one in every 12 women will be a victim of VAWG every year and one

DOI: 10.4324/9781003393160-1

in every 20 adults will be a perpetrator of such violence against women. These numbers are conservative estimates and, as noted in the report, are likely only the tip of the iceberg. As data about the number of victims each year do not exist, the NPCC report has provided estimates based on the Crime Survey for England and Wales (CSEW) data (Office for National Statistics, 2023). It is also worth saying that some police officers themselves are responsible for perpetuating violence against women. This has troubling implications for women's already low trust in the criminal justice system. For example, the 2021 murder of Sarah Everard by Met Police Officer Wayne Couzens, and Met Police Officer David Carrick, who was jailed for life in 2023 after being found guilty of multiple rapes and serious sexual assaults over a period of 17 years. I want to specify that while people of all genders can experience domestic abuse victimisation, there is a need to acknowledge power relations within a patriarchal structure whereby women and girls experience violence victimisation in particular gendered ways (Nicholson, 2019).

I do not think we *need* to list these examples to show the current extent and problem of VAWG in the UK. As I noted, the media reports and news outlets are difficult - near impossible - not to notice. However, I wanted to provide a few examples to situate this book, which is about young women's experiences of childhood domestic abuse, in the broader socio-cultural and political context of VAWG. According to the NPCC report on VAWG (National Police Chief's Council, 2024), domestic abuse is estimated to have the second highest number of victims per year (sexual harassment being the highest estimated number of victims per year). According to Women's Aid statistics (Women's Aid, 2024), over 60% of the women accessing their services have children. Yet, routes to support for children and really understanding the nuanced and complex ways that childhood experiences of domestic violence can shape children's lives throughout their lifespan are still somewhat limited.

It is well known that those who experience domestic violence in childhood are significantly impacted by these experiences, and that these experiences of violence can shape a person's sense of who they are. In the context of domestic violence in childhood, people can be impacted in ways that go far beyond bearing 'witness' to violence. However, much of the existing academic literature tends to take an interest in how children cope, factors that contribute to resilience and in identifying specific categories or demographics (such as age, gender, or severity of violence) that can help us to understand who is more likely to experience particular kinds of short- and long-term psychological, emotional and behavioural impacts of experiencing (or as it is sometimes framed, 'witnessing') domestic violence.

These are, of course, important lines of inquiry, and this knowledge can help to inform ways of supporting people in living lives that feel fulfilling and meaningful even in the aftermath of violence and trauma. However, at the time of writing this book, and when I was working on this research,

I found that there was not a huge amount of existing literature that fully captures a broad range of people's stories and experiences. I found that an over-emphasis on measuring outcomes, characteristics and traits, and a particular interest in resilience leads to an over-representation of knowledge that addresses these questions. This has implications for the kinds of knowledge generated about children who experience domestic violence in childhood, such as an assumption that resilience looks a particular way or that there is an overwhelming inevitability of 'damage' because of violence in childhood. These are troubling narratives. What I found by engaging with the qualitative research based on lived experiences was that children's lives and adults' retrospective experiences, as told by themselves, included much more nuanced and diverse accounts. This also rang true in my clinical experience as a counsellor and psychotherapist and in my own personal life experiences too.

This book is about how young adult women living in England talk about experiences of domestic violence in childhood and their transitions to young adulthood. I base this book on my doctoral research project, which I conducted between 2016 and 2020, when I interviewed ten young adult women who had experienced childhood domestic violence. The book draws on feminist psychology and a dialogical way of viewing selfhood and identity to explore how the women I interviewed narrated the 'self' and constructed a sense of self through their stories and in the relational and socio-cultural contexts within which they told their stories. The book focuses on how young women told stories of recovery and transitions to young adulthood. It pays attention to the socio-cultural contexts of young women's lives by attending to the gendered narrative resources that childhood violence and trauma can be made sense of and accounted for through stories of recovery and transitions. By taking a central interest in 'voice' – in particular, polyvocality – I examine how epistemic injustice, including testimonial injustice and hermeneutical injustice, has shaped women's histories and continues to shape how young adult women narrate childhood violence and trauma and their transitions to young adulthood. I consider how listening practices can support work toward epistemic justice, and I consider how more marginalised and less 'credible' voices get communicated and heard.

Domestic violence in childhood

Chapter 2 offers a more in-depth discussion and exploration of domestic violence in children's lives and provides context for the research this book is based on. However, to provide some grounding, I want to give a brief overview of the pervasiveness of domestic abuse, what is meant by domestic violence and abuse in the book and the extent of how it can impact children's lives in the current social, political and economic landscape. Domestic abuse refers to forms of intimate partner violence, including physical, emotional, sexual, financial and coercive control. I understand domestic abuse as characterised by pervasive, ongoing relational dynamics and a pattern of controlling and coercive behaviour rather than one-off incidents. You will notice in this book that I interchangeably use the terms 'domestic abuse', which reflects current legislation in the UK, and I use the term 'domestic violence', or more broadly, 'violence' or 'trauma'. If I refer to particular literature, I try to use terminology that reflects the language the literature uses where it feels appropriate or where it makes sense to do so. I also try to use language which reflects the language the women I spoke to used or language that feels a more accurate way of summarising experiences of violence or trauma that include domestic abuse but might include other forms of violence and abuse too. My interchangeable use of the terms 'domestic abuse' and 'domestic violence' is intentional. It is to recognise how domestic abuse is currently named in legislation and policy in the UK, and it also feels important to name it as 'violence', underpinned with the understanding that any form of abuse, coercion or control over another person *is* a form of interpersonal, systemic and structural violence.

The World Health Organization estimates that 1 in 3 women worldwide have experienced physical or sexual violence from an intimate partner or non-partner in their lifetime (World Health Organization, 2024). At the time of writing this book, the latest data on domestic abuse prevalence in England and Wales, indicated by the CSEW, estimates that 2.1 million adults experienced domestic abuse in the year ending March 2023 (Office for National Statistics, 2023). Women's Aid (2024) data shows that the most common kinds of abuse reported by people accessing services were emotional abuse (85.4%) and jealous and controlling behaviour (65.4%), with the third most common being physical abuse (52.5%). I note these statistics to give some context for the work in this book, but it should also be said that figures do say something, but they do not represent the reality of living with violence and abuse daily or the reality of what can be left behind afterwards. Also, there are limitations to gathering data only from those who report the violence or who seek formal support, as many do not report or seek formal support. Therefore, their experiences are left uncounted in these numbers.

It has been widely recognised that children are significantly impacted by their experiences of living with domestic abuse. However, up until the introduction of the Domestic Abuse Act (2021) (UK Government, 2021), which explicitly recognises and names children as direct victims of domestic abuse, children had been notably obscured from criminal law in this respect. The Westminster Government's definition of domestic abuse had previously not explicitly named children as victims. This recognition marks a step in recognising the direct impacts on children and hopefully will mark a turn to improve support provision and our understanding of the realities of how children are affected by domestic abuse.

A National Society for the Prevention of Cruelty to Children (NSPCC) prevalence study of child maltreatment in the UK suggested that approximately 25%

of young adults experienced maltreatment in childhood, including exposure to parental domestic violence (Radford et al., 2013). The NSPCC prevalence study, as far as I know, is the most widely cited and most up-to-date study that provides prevalence statistics about child exposure to domestic abuse in the UK, although this should come with the caveat that whilst it is the most up-to-date study that I can find, it is, indeed, not recent. The study did not focus on domestic abuse exclusively. However, it did identify that victimisation experiences can accumulate with age for all kinds of maltreatment and abuse, and they identified, in line with others (e.g. Finkelhor, 2018), that it is common for types of maltreatment to overlap and for children to experience multiple forms of adversity and abuse. It should be noted that the survey was relatively small, measuring the prevalence and impact of child maltreatment in a random UK representative sample of 2,160 parents/caregivers, 2,275 children and young people and 1,761 young adults using self-report measures. But what is useful is that it is one of the only prevalence studies that directly seeks children's responses, rather than adult-by-proxy, offering a potentially more accurate picture of what children directly report themselves based on their lived experiences, rather than adult reporting, which may not represent children's realities.

Domestic abuse is the most common risk factor in situations where children could be seriously harmed in England (Action for Children, 2019). Drawing on data from a sample of 39,698 women who had used Women's Aid services between 2022 and 2023 including community-based services and refuge services, Women's Aid found that most women (61.5%) had children, with an average of 1.3 children per service user, and 60.6% of these children were aged 0–10 (Women's Aid, 2024). They also found that 6.1% of women were pregnant. What this shows us is that even though there are many women who do not access specialist services, amongst those who do, most are making their way to and through services with children.

Even though legislation via the Domestic Abuse Act (2021) (UK Government, 2021) recognises children as direct victims, children and parents with children are likely to experience significant barriers when seeking formal support and safety. Women's Aid reported that less than half of refuge services could accommodate women with two children, and less than one in five could accommodate a woman with three children (Women's Aid, 2024). Community-based services offer various service types of support that differ across local authorities, meaning there is somewhat of a postcode lottery. However, the Women's Aid (2024) Audit found that only 60% of local services provide dedicated services for children and young people. This is in line with what Action for Children (2019) found in their survey of local authority service provision; they found that children face significant barriers to accessing support in at least two-thirds of local authority areas and in four of the 30 local authority areas surveyed there were no services for children and young people affected by domestic abuse at all.

Despite a wealth of evidence that shows how children are directly impacted by domestic abuse, domestic abuse has historically been understood and constructed as an issue that only adults experience. The last couple of decades of academic research has seen a shift to recognising children as 'experiencing' domestic abuse rather than simply 'witnessing' it. This shift has come alongside a gradual increase in qualitative research with children that aims to centre children's lived experiences as valuable sources of knowledge. For example, Peled (1998), Mullender et al. (2002) and Graham-Bermann and Edleson (2001) were amongst the first to speak with children themselves about their own experiences and views or centre the priorities of children. As such, slowly, children's voices in domestic violence research have become much more centralised.

This push for the centralisation of children's voices parallels a broader political and legal focus in the Global North on children's rights (*UN Convention on the Rights of the Child* (UNCRC), 1989), leading to increased interest in centring children's voices in research. Consequently, in part as a product of sustained efforts to listen to children's own sense-making and experiences, the assumption that children are passive witnesses to violence and abuse has been challenged (Åkerlund & Sandberg, 2017; Callaghan et al., 2018; Överlien & Hydén, 2009). Challenging assumptions of passivity offers alternative positions for children as being active, resilient, and both vulnerable and having the capacity to resist violence. This qualitative research has, over time, built knowledge that challenges the idea that children are both passive witnesses to domestic violence and inevitably damaged by their exposure (Överlien & Holt, 2018).

What this book does

This book is based on research I conducted where I interviewed young adult women about their experiences of childhood domestic violence. This book explores how women I interviewed narrated transitions to young adulthood and their recoveries following domestic violence in childhood. It examines how young women narrated their stories, the narrative resources that shaped their storytelling practices, and the creative narrative strategies they used to communicate tensions, ambiguities and more marginalised voices that sometimes risk becoming incommunicable or unheard. In this research, I used a qualitative feminist narrative approach, assuming that stories *do* something. It is an assumption that through stories, we construct a sense of self and communicate something about who we are and how we came to be. I hope that this book contributes something useful to readers by offering a critical and feminist exploration of gendered power structures that shape how young women tell their life stories and how they are heard. I explore how these speaking and listening practices can have implications for epistemic injustice and how we might work toward epistemic justice. I consider how speakers' voices are shaped by both personal individual biographies *and* by the socio-cultural contexts within which they speak in the aftermath of childhood domestic abuse and, more broadly, violence and trauma in childhood.

The research I explore in this book is based on research conducted in the UK, with participants all living in England at the time of the research. As such, the book is based in a UK context, and it does not intend to make claims to be generalised across cultural contexts different to the UK – England, in particular. Because of this, I draw on literature and research that is similarly centred on domestic violence in Global North and Western European cultural contexts, acknowledging that cultural, historical and political contexts hugely shape local understandings of domestic violence. This includes local understandings and practices relating to legislation and policy around violence against women, human rights and gender equity and the impacts and legacies of colonialism. I say this to be explicit that this book is a product of the culture it is written in, and it is a product of myself and my own socially located positioning as a white British woman. However, many of the themes this book addresses, around epistemic injustice, how we listen to young adult women's accounts of trauma and violence, how women might story their accounts and the entanglements of personal biographical stories with the socio-cultural contexts within which lives are lived, and stories are told, are applicable to contexts beyond the UK. As such, I hope this book will have some resonance across different Global North or Western Eurocentric cultural contexts.

This book is meant primarily for people interested in violence against women, people who are interested in domestic abuse and gender-based violence and people who are interested in thinking critically about what kinds of knowledge we value and from whom. It is intended for academics, students, practitioners, law and policymakers and anyone interested in how we listen to and hear people's stories, especially in the context of trauma and violence. It is a book centred on research, and as such, I offer reflections on theory and research practices in the context of trauma, violence and domestic abuse work.

The structure of the book

As a brief orientation to the book, this book is organised into nine chapters, which are summarised below.

Following this introductory chapter, *Chapter 2* provides an overview and critical discussion of existing literature relating to childhood accounts of domestic violence, the impacts of domestic violence and understandings of developmental transitions and change.

Chapter 3 locates this work in feminist psychology and examines the historical context that shapes how women's accounts of violence and trauma have historically and currently been discredited and why it is crucial to critically examine the epistemic practices that underpin how women are heard and the narrative practices women may use when voicing their stories.

Chapter 4 outlines Dialogical Self Theory (Hermans, 2001, 2022), which informs how I make sense of women's accounts. This chapter also provides an overview of how I conducted the research, who the participants were and how I analysed the data.

Chapters 5, 6 and 7 explore the research findings. These chapters include voice poems that I created from interview transcripts and they include extracts from transcripts. These chapters take a deeper dive into the individual participants' accounts. *Chapter 5* examines how young women narrated transitions to young adulthood. *Chapter 6* focuses on narrations of recoveries after violence in childhood. *Chapter 7* explores the creative narrative strategies women used to invite me to 'stay with' and hear the parts of their stories that might risk being marginalised or unheard.

Chapter 8 offers a reflexive account of how I listened to women's stories, proposing that embodied reflexive listening and creative artful modes of inquiry offered ways of understanding the data and understanding parts of myself, too.

Finally, *Chapter 9* draws together my concluding reflections. I consider the theoretical, methodological, and practice-based implications arising from this work and offer concluding thoughts about epistemic justice in the context of childhood domestic violence. I pay particular attention to the kinds of narrative resources that women used and how the stories they told could be both simultaneously useful and constraining. I offer concluding thoughts about how we communicate, make sense of and listen to women's stories of childhood violence.

References

Action for Children. (2019). *Patchy, piecemeal and precarious: Support for children affected by domestic abuse.* https://media.actionforchildren.org.uk/documents/patchy-piecemeal-and-precarious-support-for-children-affected-by-domestic-abuse.pdf

Åkerlund, N., & Sandberg, L. J. (2017). Children and violence interactions: Exploring intimate partner violence and children's experiences of responses. *Child Abuse Review, 26*(1), 51–62. https://doi.org/10.1002/car.2438

Callaghan, J. E. M., Alexander, J., & Fellin, L. (2018). Beyond vulnerability: Working with children who have experienced domestic violence. In L. O'Dell, C. Brownlow, & H. Bertilsdotter-Rosqvist (Eds.), *Different childhoods: Non/normative development and transgressive trajectories* (pp. 85–101). Routledge.

Finkelhor, D. (2018). Screening for adverse childhood experiences (ACEs): Cautions and suggestions. *Child Abuse & Neglect, 85*, 174–179. https://doi.org/10.1016/J.CHIABU.2017.07.016

Graham-Bermann, S. A., & Edleson, J. L. (2001). *Domestic violence in the lives of children: The future of research, intervention and social policy.* American Psychological Association.

Hermans, H. J. M. (2001). The dialogical self: Toward a theory of personal and cultural positioning. *Culture & Psychology*, 7(3), 243–281. https://doi.org/10.1177/1354067X0173001

Hermans, H. J. M. (2022). *Liberation in the face of uncertainty. A new development in dialogical self theory*. Cambridge University Press.

Lazard, L. (2020). *Sexual harassment, psychology and feminism. #MeToo, victim politics and predators in neoliberal times*. Palgrave Macmillan.

Maier, S. L. (2023). Rape victim advocates' perceptions of the #MeToo movement: Opportunities, challenges, and sustainability. *Journal of Interpersonal Violence*, 38(1–2), 336–365. https://doi.org/10.1177/08862605221081929

Mullender, A., Hague, G., Imam, U., Kelly, L., Malos, E., & Regan, L. (2002). *Children's perspectives on domestic violence*. SAGE Publications.

National Police Chief's Council. (2024). *Violence against women and girls (VAWG) national policing statement*. https://news.npcc.police.uk/resources/vteb9-ec4cx-7xgru-wufru-5vvo6

Nicholson, P. (2019). *Domestic violence and psychology. Critical perspectives on intimate partner violence and abuse* (2nd ed.). Routledge.

Office for National Statistics. (2023). *Domestic abuse prevalence and trends, England and Wales - Office for National Statistics*. https://www.ons.gov.uk/peoplepopulationandcommunity/crimeandjustice/articles/domesticabuseprevalenceandtrendsenglandandwales/yearendingmarch2023

Överlien, C., & Holt, S. (2018). Letter to the editor: Research on children experiencing domestic violence. *Journal of Family Violence*, 34(1), 65–67. https://doi.org/10.1007/s10896-018-9997-9

Överlien, C., & Hydén, M. (2009). Children's actions when experiencing domestic violence. *Childhood*, 16(4), 479–496. https://doi.org/10.1177/0907568209343757

Peled, E. (1998). The experience of living with violence for preadolescent children of battered women. *Youth & Society*, 29(4), 395–430. https://doi.org/10.1177/0044118X98029004001

Radford, L., Corral, S., Bradley, C., & Fisher, H. L. (2013). The prevalence and impact of child maltreatment and other types of victimization in the UK: Findings from a population survey of caregivers, children and young people and young adults. *Child Abuse & Neglect*, 37(10), 801–813. https://doi.org/10.1016/j.chiabu.2013.02.004

Topping, A., Hall, R., & Banfield-Nwachi, M. (2024). *Killed women count*. The Guardian. https://www.theguardian.com/uk-news/ng-interactive/2024/mar/08/killed-women-count-a-project-highlighting-the-toll-and-tragedy-of-violence-against-women-in-the-uk

UK Government. (2021). *Domestic abuse act 2021*. Domestic Abuse Act 2021. https://www.legislation.gov.uk/ukpga/2021/17/enacted

UN Convention on the Rights of the Child (UNCRC). (1989). https://www.unicef.org.uk/what-we-do/un-convention-child-rights/

Women's Aid. (2024). *The domestic abuse report 2024: The annual audit*. https://www.womensaid.org.uk/annual-audit-2024/

World Health Organization. (2024). *Violence against women*. https://www.who.int/news-room/fact-sheets/detail/violence-against-women

2
DOMESTIC VIOLENCE IN CHILDREN'S LIVES

Introduction

In this chapter, I provide a critical overview of existing research regarding what we currently know about how children experience and are affected by domestic abuse. I will then look at the literature about adulthood accounts of childhood domestic abuse. This chapter critically examines how this knowledge has come about and the potential implications of methods of knowledge generation and their epistemic underpinnings. I will also critically examine individualising discourses of 'resilience' in the aftermath of childhood adversities. Through a socio-cultural lens, I will explore what this means for how domestic abuse in childhood is understood and what divergence from normative developmental trajectories means for those whose life experiences do not align with normative ideologies, family lives and social expectations.

Children as not simply 'witnesses' to violence

You might notice that I have used the term 'children who *experience* domestic abuse' rather than children who are *exposed* or who *witness* domestic abuse. This is an intentional decision. Over the past decade, qualitative researchers have advocated for a shift of language to challenge the idea that children are passive witnesses to domestic violence and instead recognise that children are active members of families and directly involved in family dynamics where there is domestic violence (Callaghan et al., 2016; Swanston et al., 2014). For example, researchers have found that children can be directly involved by being used as a 'tool' by the abusive partner; by perpetrators using contact with children or the family court proceedings to undermine the mother–child relationship (Katz, 2016, 2022); perpetrators using the same tactics of coercive control that they use against their partner, towards the children too (Katz et al., 2020); by children directly intervening in order to protect another family member or stop or re-direct the violence (Callaghan et al., 2016; Överlien, 2017; Överlien & Hydén, 2009) or by the abusive partner using post-separation contact with the child in order to maintain control over their (ex) partner and the child(ren) (Morrison, 2015; Thiara & Humphreys, 2017). These are not the only ways that children can be directly involved, but they are some examples to show that children's experiences of violence are far more than 'witnessing' it or being 'exposed' to it.

Recognising that domestic violence is not an adult issue only and can have significant implications for children has been an important development in domestic violence research over the past two decades. As I highlighted in Chapter 1, more qualitative researchers have sought the views of children themselves. This push to centralise children's views and voices, as well as the vast evidence base showing the multiple ways in which children are affected by domestic abuse, has ultimately led to legislative recognition in UK government in the Domestic Abuse Act (2021) (UK Government, 2021) that children are direct victims if they are living with domestic abuse.

From childhood to adulthood, after domestic violence

Domestic violence can have a haunting legacy on people's lives. Domestic violence, or the impact of it, does not necessarily end when the child reaches adulthood. The person may still want to have contact with the perpetrator, or the perpetrator may insist on strategies to maintain contact that is not wanted. This section of the chapter turns attention to what we know about adults' perspectives and experiences after domestic violence in childhood. While qualitative methods are less frequently used in research with adults who experienced domestic violence in childhood, existing qualitative research highlights some important factors. For over two decades, a small number of retrospective qualitative studies have been conducted with adults who experienced domestic violence in childhood with a focus on resilience.

In 2001, Humphreys conducted a qualitative study by gathering life histories via interviews with ten adult women (aged 20–40) who had grown up with domestic violence and who were identified as living meaningful and fulfilling lives (e.g. those who were considered resilient) by workers at women's service agencies that were used as recruitment sites and by the participants themselves. Humphreys (2001) explored the biological, social, cultural and psychosocial dimensions of women's experiences, and identified themes of tension and fear that were pervasive in their lives. Importantly, Humphreys suggested that vulnerability and resilience co-existed. She found that while women lived in fear of stigma and retribution, they also maintained a sense of self and felt they lived rewarding lives.

In 2006, Anderson and Danis used an approach that sought to generate a theory based on information gathered by interviewing 12 adult women (aged 22–54). They used a grounded theory approach to explore women's views about their experiences of growing up with domestic violence (father-to-mother violence) and their sense of what had helped them to cope (Anderson & Danis refer to this as resilience). Their findings highlight that resilience was rooted in their resistance to their father's perpetration of violence against their mother and the consequences of their father's violence. Anderson and Danis (2006) highlighted that the women they interviewed used several protective strategies that served to withstand and oppose their sense of powerlessness because of their father's violence. Their conclusions highlight the importance of acknowledging that resistance and vulnerabilities can and do co-exist. They show that looking at the operation of power and resistance against oppression can help highlight resistance strategies in the face of violence.

Suzuki et al. (2008) interviewed two men and eight women, aged 23–35, about the protective factors or resiliencies that they felt contributed to their adaptive outcomes (or resiliency) after childhood domestic violence. Their analysis included themes that covered individual, external and family factors, such as social support and important adult figures in childhood, closeness to someone in family of origin or closeness with one parent, accepting imperfections of the family and ability to regulate emotions, learn from the past and pursue goals. Some aspects of these findings can also be read in O'Brien et al.'s (2013) study. They used a case study approach to interview six women (aged 18–39) about their recounted memories of childhood domestic violence. Key coping strategies they identified included establishing a safe retreat outside the family home and having a supportive relationship outside the family home. They proposed these are key aspects that help adult women 'move on' and lead a 'rewarding' adult life. They also identified several other coping strategies participants recounted that helped them to deal with the isolation and depression that they experienced, such as attempts to stop the abuse and attempts to block out the abuse.

In a turn to focus on men, Gonzales et al. (2012) focused on men's resiliency. They interviewed 12 adult men who experienced domestic violence in childhood and who they identified via initial screening questionnaires as 'non-violent', 'successful' and 'resilient'. They explored the contextual factors that contributed to the resilience of the men. They found that men identified factors such as having key safe relationships with caring adults and a safe haven outside of the home, using positive coping strategies like extracurricular activities and sports, and gaining professional and personal achievements. They draw attention to the need to pay attention to how gender norms shape people's coping strategies and the need for a more diverse approach to considering what constitutes resilience after childhood domestic violence.

More recently, Levell's (2022) research with men who experienced domestic violence in childhood engages with the intersections of race, gender and class as they shape men's lives and identities. Specifically, she examined intersections of domestic violence and abuse (DVA) with other forms of violence that are specific to the lives of men who are gang-involved or on-road, and who have grown up with DVA. Her work evidences the complex ways in which the men she interviewed navigate violence, vulnerability and identity. Levell's engagement with the tensions of vulnerability and violence is important. While it is well known that DVA often occurs alongside other forms of family violence and adversities (Lamers-Winkelman et al., 2012), these intersections are not often critically examined.

What is salient about Levell's (2022) work is that she demonstrates the importance of staying with and examining tensions evident in men's accounts. A unique contribution of this work is the gendered analysis of men's accounts. Levell argues that boys are very excluded; for instance, they have limited access to refuge spaces, and they tend to be framed as posing a threat from a young age, particularly if they are Black. This is a crucial and much-needed gendered and intersectional analysis in DVA work (Damant et al., 2008; Sokoloff & Dupont, 2005). Levell invites readers to resist individualising conceptualisations and practices, which can be pathologising and deterministic. She invites readers to stay with the tensions these men navigate by simultaneously holding vulnerability and violence.

Lastly, Dumont and Lessard (2020) explored the experiences and perspectives of young adults with a broader focus on meanings assigned to childhood experiences of domestic violence rather than specifically on resilience or coping, offering a significant addition to the literature. They focused on Canadian young adults (aged 18–25) meaning-making in relation to childhood experiences of domestic violence. Their work diverges from existing qualitative literature on young adults as it does not centre around coping or resilience. Specifically, they suggest that development consists of multiple factors for young adults over the life course. Their findings offer a useful springboard for the work in this book, indicating that developmental transitions for those who experience domestic violence in childhood can be understood as more nuanced, complex, individual and relational than most existing literature suggests.

A prevailing focus on resilience?

My reading is that some of the above studies focus *only* on resilience and coping (e.g. Humphreys, 2001; O'Brien et al., 2013; Suzuki et al., 2008). A strength-based focus on resilience can be helpful. It is, of course, useful to consider what helps people to cope and survive through violence in childhood. However, this is also troubling. An underpinning assumption that some people evidence resilience and others do not is problematic. It is problematic to assume that there are universal and narrow ways to assess and measure resilience *and* that an individual can be defined as either resilient or not when resilience is known to be fluid, context-dependant and dynamic.

Often (but not always), a criterion for participating in the above studies has been that the participant demonstrates they are in a healthy, non-violent relationship, their scores on wellbeing questionnaires are considered healthy or within the 'normal' range and they identify the participants as living fulfilling, rewarding or successful lives. These ideas about wellness, success and resilience after childhood domestic violence are, in some ways, hopeful. Many people *do* live these kinds of lives, and in the face of some prevailing and negative societal messaging about violence victimisation equating to 'damage' or even violence in adulthood for some, acknowledging stories like this is fundamental. However, my concern is that these ideas reproduce the idea that adult outcomes based on childhood experiences can only be understood through a binary either–or lens (e.g. successful or unsuccessful, resilient or not).

As evidenced by some of the above existing qualitative studies (e.g. Anderson & Danis, 2006; Dumont & Lessard, 2020; Levell, 2022), it is vital to engage with the concept of resilience in a nuanced way when understanding the lived realities of childhood domestic violence. A focus on resilience or coping limits the space for people to express and for listeners to understand how transitions to adulthood are experienced beyond factors contributing to resilience or coping, or indeed, expressions of survival and coping that do not align with dominant ways of understanding survival or strength.

Qualitative research supports the production of knowledge that is more nuanced and aligned with lived experiences, but there is still a dominance of quantitatively driven evidence, which I referred to at the beginning of this chapter, which identifies the long-lasting outcomes that exposure to domestic abuse can result in. Such research has centred on children lacking emotional regulation skills, the capacity to build peer relationships and the capacity to achieve 'well' in school or later life (Holt et al., 2008; Meltzer et al., 2009). These conclusions reflect a deficit model of development, a focus on what is *lacking* and what is *wrong* according to normative standards, despite the many researchers who have included the voices of children themselves and suggest alternative positions for children as agentic, resourceful and resistant (Frances & Carter, 2023; Överlien & Holt, 2018).

In this chapter so far, I have critically examined existing literature about how children can be impacted by domestic violence in childhood, how children experience domestic violence and how adults are affected and make sense of these experiences retrospectively. In the research with adults, there is a particular interest in adult experiences where these adults have identified themselves or been identified by researchers or clinicians as 'resilient', 'non-violent', or perhaps underpinning these assumptions is a sense that they have come out of enduring violence 'well' and might have something valuable to offer researchers. The literature I have discussed importantly acknowledges that people's lives can be profoundly shaped, and people can be significantly harmed by childhood domestic violence. However, much of this evidence fails to critically examine underpinning discourses. This evidence can be understood as situated within the psy-disciplines (Rose, 2008) (e.g. psychology, psychiatry or psychotherapy). I discuss this further in the sections that follow in this chapter.

Thinking beyond 'adverse childhood experiences'

Domestic abuse is considered an 'adverse childhood experience' (ACE). In the late 1990s, a well-known series of studies examined the combined effects of multiple negative early life experiences, otherwise known as ACEs. The first of the ACE studies was conducted by Felitti and colleagues (Felitti et al., 1998). They investigated the relationship between exposure to childhood adversities, including emotional, physical or sexual abuse, and household 'dysfunction'[1] to disease, health status and health-risk behaviour in adulthood. They conducted their study in a Health Appraisal Clinic in San Diego. They mailed a questionnaire to 13,494 adults who had attended the clinic and completed a standardised medical evaluation. The questionnaire asked participants to self-report about ACEs and their health-related behaviours and problems. They received 9,508 responses. They studied seven categories of ACEs. These were psychological, physical or sexual abuse; violence against mother; or living with household members who were substance abusers, mentally ill or suicidal or ever imprisoned. They then compared the number of self-reported ACEs with the health behaviours and problems reported and analysed the self-report questionnaire data alongside information gathered by the Health Appraisal Clinic's standardised medical evaluation.

One of the major findings from this study is still very often cited now, especially in trauma-informed care literature. Felitti et al. (1998) found that more than half of respondents reported at least one category of ACE, and one-fourth reported two or more categories of childhood exposures. They found that people who had experienced four or more categories of childhood exposure, compared to those who had experienced none, had a 4- to 12-fold increased risk of adulthood health difficulties, including risks for alcoholism, drug abuse, depression and suicide attempts. The number of categories of adverse childhood exposures also showed an increased presence of physical health conditions, including heart disease, lung disease and cancer. In short, these findings suggest that experiencing adversities in childhood is linked to poor health outcomes in adulthood, and the more adversities a child experiences, the more likely it is that they will experience these poor health outcomes in adulthood that are strongly linked to risk factors associated with the leading causes of death in adults. Using this evidence, Felitti and colleagues produced a 10-item questionnaire (Adverse Childhood Experiences Questionnaire, known as ACE-Q) that could be completed and then scored. Higher scores indicated exposure to more types of childhood adversity and suggested a greater likelihood of poor health outcomes. This scoring logic has since been critiqued as being 'relatively crude' (Anda et al., 2020, p. 293). It can be potentially misused and misappropriated as screening or diagnostic tools to assess the risk of negative health and social problems and determine treatment pathways despite little peer-reviewed research to support this use of the ACE scoring system (Anda et al., 2020). Despite these problems, there is still a movement toward using such a scoring system to screen for childhood trauma (Anda et al., 2020).

Domestic violence is one of the ACEs listed by Felliti and colleagues, or, as it was named in the study, 'violence against mother'. While I do not want to portray a damning picture of 'damage' as if this is the only inevitable outcome, I do want to highlight the wealth of research that shows the numerous ways in which research tells us children are impacted by living with domestic abuse. For example, research shows that experiencing domestic abuse can have significant impacts on the mental health of children, and this can last long into adulthood (Hughes et al., 2017). It can impact their attachment functioning (Fusco, 2017; Gustafsson et al., 2017; Levendosky et al., 2011; Sousa et al., 2011), the potential for future involvement in violent relationships (Holmes, 2013) and means these children are more likely to experience difficulties with emotion regulation and peer relationships (Easterbrooks et al., 2018; Fainsilber Katz et al., 2016).

These studies clearly show that the impacts of childhood domestic violence are largely negative. These kinds of outcomes are widely recognised, but it should also be noted that it is mostly based on quantitative evidence that relies on secondary reporting – that is, it relies on numerical data that is provided by adults (such as clinicians or caregivers) rather than lived experiences as told by children themselves. These methods are common for this kind of research that is interested in generalising across populations, that is interested in trends and that is interested in understanding outcomes and long-term trajectories of particular sub-populations based on categories and demographics. This approach is not necessarily problematic. However, these methodologies only capture a partial and incomplete story and, importantly, miss out lived experiences as voiced by people themselves.

Additionally, there is a need for a critical examination of the assumptions that underpin this research. As Levell (2022) notes, 'There is an air of "adversity-as-destiny" that is inherent with a checklist that seeks to generalize complex human contexts based on simplistic cumulative score' (p. 29). Levell accurately summarises the troubling way that ACE scores can act as an additive way of generalising lived experiences of violence that are much more nuanced than can be captured in a score. Simultaneously, ACE scores tell a very singular, narrow story. The implied assumption is that increased adversity equals poorer chances in life and poorer outcomes. This does not enable space for alternative stories, or experiences that contain resilience, resistance and all kinds of ways of living with, living through and making sense of domestic violence.

Resilient brains and resilient people: is this really what it's about?

Most of the research shows how childhood adversities raise the risk of poorer outcomes for children, but more so for children who experience multiple adversities as opposed to one. This is perhaps unsurprising. If you are familiar with literature about how the brain and body respond to stressful or traumatic experiences, then you will know that stress responses can be considered both a physiological and psychosocial process, which can be experienced differently depending on individual and social or environmental factors. This is commonly known as the 'Fight, Flight, Freeze or Fawn' response as a physiological threat response. Much of this evidence is rooted in the physiology of the nervous system, leading us to a way of thinking about stress responses and resilience as things that are located within individual brains (and bodies) – this is what I refer to here as a neuroscientific discourse of the 'resilient brain' as a way of understanding resilience after enduring trauma and in the face of adversity (Macvarish et al., 2015; Rose, 2010; Wastell & White, 2012).

The ACE study findings are aligned with a body of trauma literature that clearly shows a link between early life stress, psychological trauma and poorer physical health outcomes (López-Martínez et al., 2018; Maschi et al., 2013; Zarse et al., 2019). However, there are valid critiques of a purely biologising and medicalising way of understanding the impacts of psychological trauma because of how this can be reductionist and fail to attend to the human experience more holistically and psychosocially. In my view, knowledge about how the physical health of bodies can be affected is still important. An anti-Cartesian logic (Launeanu & Kwee, 2018), where mind and body are considered not as separate entities but as part of one whole system, is a useful lens that demonstrates bodymind systems can be affected by what we experience. This is supported by many trauma writers and practitioners who advocate for somatic psychotherapies and embodiment-oriented ways of working that can support people to heal and recover after trauma (Emerson & Hopper, 2011; Ogden & Minton, 2000; Rothschild, 2017).

My intention is not to suggest that neuroscientific evidence is not helpful. As a psychotherapy practitioner myself, I find neuroscience very helpful, in part, in helping myself and clients to make sense of how stress and trauma may have had a lasting impact, and how wise and resourceful bodies and brains can be in keeping us alert to potential threats and doing what we can do to keep ourselves safe when we sense danger. However, minds and bodies exist in socio-cultural contexts, and this neuroscientific lens becomes limited if it is the *only* way we understand stress responses and human resilience after trauma (Burman, 2017; Featherstone et al., 2014; Rose, 2010; Wastell & White, 2012). This neuroscience discourse has even been critiqued from within neuroscience itself. For instance, the understanding that different regions of the brain are responsible for different functions (known as localisation) has been argued to be limited and outdated, and psychologists have questioned the extent to which we understand regions of the brain (Uttal, 2011).

While we are still learning more and more about the brain, as technology advances and knowledge expands, the dominant focus on neuroscience remains fairly unchallenged in mainstream practice, meaning that ideas around the 'resilient brain' continue to be pervasive. This pervasive presence continues to reproduce assumptions that resilience and wellness in adulthood are individual traits and, therefore, unrelated to and not connected with social and relational contexts (Gill & Scharff, 2011; Rose, 2010).

This dominant individualising framework about wellness and resilience after childhood adversities erases the examination and role of socially located power, privilege and oppression, which we know intersects profoundly with domestic violence and other kinds of childhood trauma. For example, we know that household poverty, more often than not, affects families who experience other adversities, such as parental domestic violence and poor mental health (Adjei et al., 2022). Additionally, racism and racial discrimination can contribute to and compound health inequalities (Wallace et al., 2016) and can intersect with childhood experiences of domestic violence in impactful ways (Levell, 2022). As such, it is crucial to attend to the social and structural systems that impact health inequalities and health outcomes and to challenge and resist an individualising way of thinking about resilience after trauma.

The question of what makes children and adults resilient following exposure to domestic violence threads through much of the literature (for example, see Anderson & Bang, 2012; Howell & Miller-Graff, 2014; Narayan et al., 2018). Consequently, characteristics such as age and gender, and factors such as severity of violence, sibling order and attachment functioning are treated as categories through which to assess impact, resilience and outcomes (for example, see Holt et al., 2008; Sousa et al., 2011). Insisting on a categorical approach to resilience (e.g. you are either resilient or not) is very unlikely to reflect the lived realities of people who experience violence. Categorising outcomes can be seen as a mechanism of flattening complexity and assuming that resilience is something that is inherently present or absent within an individual. As such, a focus on coping and resilience *only* is a narrow lens to look through when making efforts to understand the lives of those who experienced domestic violence in childhood.

There is an acceptance among resilience scholars that resilience is not an either/or trait, and that it exists on a continuum and is likely to present differently depending on factors such as context, individual differences, access to resources and individual history (Southwick et al., 2014). One of the main differences between some ideas about resilience is that it is either an assumption that a person has resilient traits (a person-centred model), or that resilience is a dynamic process that is subject to change across different times and places (a relational process-based model). There is little agreement on what makes people resilient in the face of adversity, but in the context of domestic violence, qualitative research suggests that families can be both a reason for adverse experiences and can also potentially provide protective factors based on some family relationships. For example, supportive family relationships, such as grandparents (Gottzén & Sandberg, 2019) and siblings (Åkerlund, 2017; Callaghan et al., 2016), and rebuilding a positive and supportive mother–child relationship (Katz, 2015) after domestic violence can support children to recover and act as protective factors.

A persistent focus on outcomes, particularly those that are considered 'pathological', has a particular function. It uses an individualising lens, positioning families or individuals as responsible for their own struggles and removing the responsibility of the state to change the social and economic inequalities that often underpin 'private' difficulties of families, such as poverty, gender-based inequalities, domestic abuse, substance use problems and mental illness (Burman, 2017; Edwards, 2002). Viewing domestic violence through an outcome-focused and individualised lens presents some troubling narrative frameworks for children and adults to make sense of their life experiences. There exists a narrative framework of outcomes that paints a picture of a non-negotiable linear trajectory where the endpoint or outcome does not look hopeful. This homogenisation of outcomes is problematic and works against a multidimensional and relational way of understanding how domestic violence in childhood is experienced.

This section of the chapter has explored the relatively small amount of qualitative research spanning across the last couple of decades that has examined the experiences of adults who experienced domestic violence as children. This research points to the importance of centring lived experiences. However, biologising and individualising assumptions about development, resilience and distress are evident even in current research about the impacts of domestic violence on children, which appears to privilege outcome-based essentialising approaches that leave an overarching message that exposure to violence leaves lasting damage by interfering with and disrupting 'normal' brain development (Thomason & Marusak, 2017). Underpinning this 'resilient brain' discourse (Burman, 2017) is a dominant individualising, sometimes-biologising understanding of distress, resilience and identity. As feminist psychologists have argued, this biomedical discourse dominates as it has the capacity and power to construct a particular version of 'truth' and reality that is bolstered and upheld by the economic, political and institutional power of medicine and science (Lafrance & McKenzie-Mohr, 2013).

The transition from childhood to adulthood in the context of childhood domestic violence is a central interest of this book. Therefore, in the following section of this chapter, I will outline why I see this transition as important for those who grow up with domestic violence, and I will outline a socio-cultural theorisation of change and transitions that informs this book.

Change and transitions: a socio-cultural perspective

Childhood development towards adulthood can be viewed as a transition. Some assumptions, in part, shaped by developmental psychology offer rigid and normative ideas about what developmental transitions should look like. For example, in Western Eurocentric cultural contexts, these markers might include entering new phases of life, such as work, employment, further education and leaving childhood homes, which are socially and culturally understood markers of becoming an adult. While adulthood and childhood are typically understood and socially and culturally constructed to be separate phases in the lifespan (Burman, 2017; James & Prout, 2015), it can also be argued that age markers do not easily define the boundary between childhood and adulthood (Valentine, 2003; Zittoun, 2007). Efforts to distinguish childhood and adulthood have been considered arbitrary, or it has been argued that examining these different life 'stages' requires a more nuanced, culturally located and individually oriented approach (Furlong, 2009).

However, these markers are not generalisable transition points, even within the cultural contexts they claim to represent. These normative markers routinely exclude those whose lives do not follow these biographical paths, and they reproduce age-based norms when, arguably, the borders between all life phases are 'less age-dependent' (Furlong, 2009, p. 11) and require a more located and nuanced view that accounts for ongoing change and fluidity. Conceptualising childhood as a stage in human development has been critiqued among critical developmental psychologists and widely among sociologists (Archard, 2004; Burman, 2017) because rigid developmental assumptions tell a story of linearity about childhood, which is not globally applicable, nor applicable to the multiplicities of lived experiences even within local cultural contexts. Childhood scholars have argued that dominant age-based ways of distinguishing 'child' and 'adult' (re)produce the idea that childhood is separate from adulthood and disrupts the kind of fluidity and continuity that can characterise developmental transitions (Burman, 2017; Walkerdine, 1993). Consequently, these dominant assumptions shape discursive grounds for making sense of those whose lives have diverged from these normative assumptions.

As I discussed earlier in this chapter, in a domestic violence context, these normative developmental assumptions include that exposure to violence interferes with and disrupts 'normal' brain development (Carpenter &

Stacks, 2009; Perry et al., 1995; Thomason & Marusak, 2017) and that children's social and emotional development and skills will be negatively affected as a result of living with domestic violence (Carpenter & Stacks, 2009; Holt et al., 2008). These types of universalising and homogenising assumptions about children's lives are troubling in relation to knowledge construction and social discourse (O'Dell et al., 2018). Different childhoods – in other words, childhoods that diverge from dominant normative understandings of children's development and normative family life – tend to be pathologised and positioned as 'other' (Burman, 2017; Walkerdine, 1993).

Processes of change can be unsettling, destabilising and uncertain. In this book, I draw on Tania Zittoun's (2007, 2008) conceptualisation of transitions to understand transitions from a socio-cultural lens and shift away from a typical age and stage-based lens that tends to focus on adulthood as the outcome and change as fixed and binary. Zittoun considers that transitions consist of many aspects, including those that are individual to a person's biography and life, and those that are shaped by our frames of reference (otherwise known as socio-cultural resources). These social and cultural resources could include family narratives or socio-cultural norms, for instance. Transitions can be understood as periods of change at any time in life, which may involve acquiring new knowledge and, consequently, different ways of making meaning out of what has happened. Processes of change and transition, according to Zittoun, can be destabilising and uncertain, and they can also offer opportunities for growth and transformation as we encounter possibilities to reconstruct and re-develop our sense of who we are. Zittoun's socio-cultural theorisation of transitions informs this work, understanding transitions as socio-culturally located processes that involve multiple fluid periods of change, the construction and reconstruction of knowledge and identity and the ongoing process of meaning-making through symbolic resources.

Summary

This chapter has explored the developing field of knowledge surrounding experiences of domestic violence in childhood. I have highlighted the valuable qualitative research that has significantly informed the evidence base about childhood experiences of domestic violence, where both children and adults have been consulted about their lived experiences. However, the study of domestic violence in childhood has been largely dominated by deficit-oriented and predominantly quantitative methods. Consequently, children and families who experience adversities, including domestic violence, are often positioned in problematic ways through social, clinical and academic discourses (Överlien & Holt, 2018).

The impacts and outcomes of childhood domestic violence are not always predictable in adulthood, and existing research has not sufficiently paid attention to how individuals make sense of their present-day selves and relationships through the lens of their childhood experiences. However, two recent studies offer important analytic reflections. Levell's (2022) work with adult men who experienced childhood domestic violence points to the need for a gendered analysis and examination of socio-cultural factors that shape adulthood accounts after childhood domestic violence. Levell (2022) draws attention to the need to stay with the tensions that men navigate by holding both vulnerability and violence simultaneously. Additionally, Dumont and Lessard (2020) explored the life courses of adults who experienced childhood domestic violence. They highlighted a need for researchers to engage with nuance and specifically that young adults construct meanings around violence that are shaped by the context of their individual lives (e.g. school, work or friendship). Therefore, a gendered and contextual analysis is necessary.

It is necessary to recognise the harm caused by adverse experiences, but the sole use of outcomes evidence as the only lens through which to view and predict outcomes is individualising and rooted in a pathologising way of thinking. Although researchers have challenged discourses of inevitable damage, outcomes evidence still holds power. The 'myth of objectivity' (Haraway, 1988) and the epistemological power of 'scientific knowledge' (Rose, 1985) can help to explain why such evidence tends to be privileged. This chapter has critically examined the underpinning knowledge systems that inform what kinds of evidence are held up as valuable. In the context of childhood domestic violence, I have argued that the dominance of psy-discourses that are presented as scientific truths (Marecek & Lafrance, 2021) provides limiting knowledge about children's trajectories to adulthood after domestic violence. Processes of change can be unsettling, destabilising and uncertain. However, theories about development are situated in cultural contexts and shaped by historical and social discourse. Knowledge constructed from 'psy-expertise' (Klein & Mills, 2017) shapes social and academic discourse that normalises and biologises human development as a natural linear stage-based and age-based process, and as such, may not enable understandings of change and transition that are non-normative, divergent or told in alternative ways.

In the chapter that follows, I consider what feminist psychology can do for this work, and I offer a more in-depth discussion of why epistemic justice and the gendered socio-cultural contexts that shape the epistemic injustices women often face when talking about violence and trauma are crucial to attend to.

Note

1 'Dysfunction' is a term the researchers used in this study, and it was a term more routinely used at this time. It refers to some of the seven categories of adverse childhood experiences they studied (psychological, physical or sexual abuse; violence against mother or living with household members who were substance abusers, mentally ill or suicidal or ever imprisoned).

References

Adjei, N. K., Schlüter, D. K., Straatmann, V. S., Melis, G., Fleming, K. M., McGovern, R., Howard, L. M., Kaner, E., Wolfe, I., & Taylor-Robinson, D. C. (2022). Impact of poverty and family adversity on adolescent health: A multi-trajectory analysis using the UK Millennium Cohort Study. *The Lancet Regional Health - Europe, 13*. https://doi.org/10.1016/J.LANEPE.2021.100279

Åkerlund, N. (2017). Caring or vulnerable children? Sibling relationships when exposed to intimate partner violence. *Children & Society, 31*(6), 475–485. https://doi.org/10.1111/chso.12215

Anda, R. F., Porter, L. E., & Brown, D. W. (2020). Inside the adverse childhood experience score: Strengths, limitations, and misapplications. *American Journal of Preventive Medicine, 59*(2), 293–295. https://doi.org/10.1016/j.amepre.2020.01.009

Anderson, K. M., & Bang, E. J. (2012). Assessing PTSD and resilience for females who during childhood were exposed to domestic violence. *Child and Family Social Work, 17*(1), 55–65. https://doi.org/10.1111/j.1365-2206.2011.00772.x

Anderson, K. M., & Danis, F. S. (2006). Adult daughters of battered women: Resistance and resilience in the face of danger. *Affilia, 21*(4), 419–432. https://doi.org/10.1177/0886109906292130

Archard, D. (2004). *Children: Rights and childhood* (2nd ed.). Routledge.

Burman, E. (2017). *Deconstructing developmental psychology* (3rd ed.). Routledge.

Callaghan, J. E. M., Alexander, J. H., Sixsmith, J., & Fellin, L. C. (2016). Children's experiences of domestic violence and abuse: Siblings' accounts of relational coping. *Clinical Child Psychology and Psychiatry, 21*(4), 649–668. https://doi.org/10.1177/1359104515620250

Carpenter, G. L., & Stacks, A. M. (2009). Developmental effects of exposure to intimate partner violence in early childhood: A review of the literature. *Children and Youth Services Review, 31*(8), 831–839. https://doi.org/10.1016/J.CHILDYOUTH.2009.03.005

Damant, D., Lapierre, S., Kouraga, A., Fortin, A., Hamelin-Brabant, L., Lavergne, C., & Lessard, G. (2008). Taking child abuse and mothering into account: Intersectional feminism as an alternative for the study of domestic violence. *Affilia, 23*(2), 123–133. https://doi.org/10.1177/0886109908314321

Dumont, A., & Lessard, G. (2020). Young adults exposed to intimate partner violence in childhood: The qualitative meanings of this experience. *Journal of Family Violence, 35*, 781–792. https://doi.org/10.1007/s10896-019-00100-z

Easterbrooks, M. A., Katz, R. C., Kotake, C., Stelmach, N. P., & Chaudhuri, J. H. (2018). Intimate partner violence in the first 2 years of life: Implications for toddlers' behavior regulation. *Journal of Interpersonal Violence, 33*(7), 1192–1214. https://doi.org/10.1177/0886260515614562

Edwards, R. (2002). *Children, home, and school regulation, autonomy or connection?* Routledge.

Emerson, D., & Hopper, E. (2011). *Overcoming trauma through yoga: Reclaiming your body*. North Atlantic Books.

Fainsilber Katz, L., Stettler, N., & Gurtovenko, K. (2016). Traumatic stress symptoms in children exposed to intimate partner violence: The role of parent emotion socialization and children's emotion regulation abilities. *Social Development, 25*(1), 47–65. https://doi.org/10.1111/sode.12151

Featherstone, B., Morris, K., & White, S. (2014). A marriage made in hell: Early intervention meets child protection. *British Journal of Social Work, 44*(7), 1735–1749. https://doi.org/10.1093/bjsw/bct052

Felitti, V. J., Anda, R. F., Nordenberg, D., Williamson, D. F., Spitz, A. M., Edwards, V., Koss, M. P., & Marks, J. S. (1998). Relationship of childhood abuse and household dysfunction to many of the leading causes of death in adults: The adverse childhood experiences (ACE) study. *American Journal of Preventive Medicine*, 14(4), 245–258. https://doi.org/10.1016/S0749-3797(98)00017-8

Frances, T., & Carter, G. (2023). Negotiating power, choice and agency: Working towards centralising children's voices in the domestic violence and abuse intervention evidence-base. In J. Taylor & E. Bates (Eds.), *Children and adolescents' experiences of violence at home: Current theory, research and practitioner insights*. Routledge.

Furlong, A. (2009). *Handbook of youth and young adulthood: New perspectives and agendas*. Routledge.

Fusco, R. A. (2017). Socioemotional problems in children exposed to intimate partner violence: Mediating effects of attachment and family supports. *Journal of Interpersonal Violence*, 32(16), 2515–2532. https://doi.org/10.1177/0886260515593545

Gill, R., & Scharff, C. (2011). *New femininities: Postfeminism, neoliberalism, and subjectivity*. Palgrave Macmillan.

Gonzales, G., Chronister, K. M., Linville, D., & Knoble, N. B. (2012). Experiencing parental violence: A qualitative examination of adult men's resilience. *Psychology of Violence*, 2(1), 90–103. https://doi.org/10.1037/a0026372

Gottzén, L., & Sandberg, L. (2019). Creating safe atmospheres? Children's experiences of grandparents' affective and spatial responses to domestic violence. *Children's Geographies*, 17(5), 514–526. https://doi.org/10.1080/14733285.2017.1406896

Gustafsson, H. C., Brown, G. L., Mills-Koonce, W. R., & Cox, M. J. (2017). Intimate partner violence and children's attachment representations during middle childhood. *Journal of Marriage and Family*, 79(3), 865–878. https://doi.org/10.1111/jomf.12388

Haraway, D. (1988). Situated knowledges: The science question in feminism and the privilege of partial perspective. *Feminist Studies*, 14(3), 575. https://doi.org/10.2307/3178066

Holmes, M. R. (2013). Aggressive behavior of children exposed to intimate partner violence: An examination of maternal mental health, maternal warmth and child maltreatment. *Child Abuse & Neglect*, 37(8), 520–530. https://doi.org/10.1016/J.CHIABU.2012.12.006

Holt, S., Buckley, H., & Whelan, S. (2008). The impact of exposure to domestic violence on children and young people: A review of the literature. *Child Abuse & Neglect*, 32(8), 797–810. https://doi.org/10.1016/J.CHIABU.2008.02.004

Howell, K. H., & Miller-Graff, L. E. (2014). Protective factors associated with resilient functioning in young adulthood after childhood exposure to violence. *Child Abuse & Neglect*, 38(12), 1985–1994. https://doi.org/10.1016/J.CHIABU.2014.10.010

Hughes, K., Bellis, M. A., Hardcastle, K. A., Sethi, D., Butchart, A., Mikton, C., Jones, L., & Dunne, M. P. (2017). The effect of multiple adverse childhood experiences on health: a systematic review and meta-analysis. *The Lancet. Public Health*, 2(8), 356–366. https://doi.org/10.1016/S2468-2667(17)30118-4

Humphreys, C. (2001). Growing up in a violent home: The lived experience of daughters of battered women. *Journal of Family Nursing*, 7(3), 244–260. https://doi.org/10.1177/107484070100700303

James, A., & Prout, A. (2015). *Constructing and reconstructing childhood: Contemporary issues in the sociological study of childhood* (2nd ed.). Routledge.

Katz, E. (2015). Domestic violence, children's agency and mother-child relationships: Towards a more advanced model. *Children & Society*, 29(1), 69–79. https://doi.org/10.1111/chso.12023

Katz, E. (2016). Beyond the physical incident model: How children living with domestic violence are harmed by and resist regimes of coercive control. *Child Abuse Review*, 25(1), 46–59. https://doi.org/10.1002/car.2422

Katz, E. (2022). *Coercive control in children's and mothers' lives*. Oxford University Press.

Katz, E., Nikupeteri, A., & Laitinen, M. (2020). When coercive control continues to harm children: Post-separation fathering, stalking and domestic violence. *Child Abuse Review*, 29(4), 310–324. https://doi.org/10.1002/CAR.2611

Klein, E., & Mills, C. (2017). Psy-expertise, therapeutic culture and the politics of the personal in development. *Third World Quarterly*, 38(9), 1990–2008. https://doi.org/10.1080/01436597.2017.1319277

Lafrance, M. N., & McKenzie-Mohr, S. (2013). The DSM and its lure of legitimacy. *Feminism & Psychology*, 23(1), 119–140. https://doi.org/10.1177/0959353512467974

Lamers-Winkelman, F., Willemen, A. M., & Visser, M. (2012). Adverse childhood experiences of referred children exposed to intimate partner violence: Consequences for their wellbeing. *Child Abuse & Neglect*, 36(2), 166–179. https://doi.org/10.1016/J.CHIABU.2011.07.006

Launeanu, M., & Kwee, J. L. (2018). A non-dualistic and existential perspective on understanding and treating disordered eating. In H. L. McBride & J. L. Kwee (Eds.), *Embodiment and eating disorders: Theory, research, prevention, and treatment* (pp. 35–52). Routledge.

Levell, J. (2022). *Boys, childhood, domestic abuse and gang involvement*. Bristol University Press.

Levendosky, A. A., Bogat, G. A., & Huth-Bocks, A. C. (2011). The influence of domestic violence on the development of the attachment relationship between mother and young child. *Psychoanalytic Psychology*, 28(4), 512–527. https://doi.org/10.1037/a0024561

López-Martínez, A. E., Serrano-Ibáñez, E. R., Ruiz-Párraga, G. T., Gómez-Pérez, L., Ramírez-Maestre, C., & Esteve, R. (2018). Physical health consequences of interpersonal trauma: A systematic review of the role of psychological variables. *Trauma Violence Abuse*, 19(3), 305–322. https://doi.org/10.1177/1524838016659488

Macvarish, J., Lee, E., & Lowe, P. (2015). Neuroscience and family policy: What becomes of the parent? *Critical Social Policy*, 35(2), 248–269. https://doi.org/10.1177/0261018315574019

Marecek, J., & Lafrance, M. N. (2021). Editorial introduction: The politics of psychological suffering. *Feminism & Psychology*, 31(1), 3–18. https://doi.org/10.1177/0959353521989537

Maschi, T., Baer, J., Morrissey, M. B., & Moreno, C. (2013). The aftermath of childhood trauma on late life mental and physical health. *Traumatology*, 19(1), 49–64. https://doi.org/10.1177/1534765612437377

Meltzer, H., Doos, L., Vostanis, P., Ford, T., & Goodman, R. (2009). The mental health of children who witness domestic violence. *Child & Family Social Work*, 14(4), 491–501. https://doi.org/10.1111/j.1365-2206.2009.00633.x

Morrison, F. (2015). 'All over now?' The ongoing relational consequences of domestic abuse through children's contact arrangements. *Child Abuse Review*, 24(4), 274–284. https://doi.org/10.1002/car.2409

Narayan, A. J., Rivera, L. M., Bernstein, R. E., Harris, W. W., & Lieberman, A. F. (2018). Positive childhood experiences predict less psychopathology and stress in pregnant women with childhood adversity: A pilot study of the benevolent childhood experiences (BCEs) scale. *Child Abuse & Neglect, 78*, 19–30. https://doi.org/10.1016/j.chiabu.2017.09.022

O'Brien, K. L., Cohen, L., Pooley, J. A., & Taylor, M. F. (2013). Lifting the domestic violence cloak of silence: Resilient Australian women's reflected memories of their childhood experiences of witnessing domestic violence. *Journal of Family Violence, 28*(1), 95–108. https://doi.org/10.1007/s10896-012-9484-7

O'Dell, L., Brownlow, C., & Bertilsdotter Rosqvist, H. (2018). *Different childhoods: Non/normative development and transgressive trajectories.* Routledge.

Ogden, P., & Minton, K. (2000). Sensorimotor psychotherapy. *Traumatology, 6*(3), 149–173. https://doi.org/10.1177/153476560000600302

Överlien, C. (2017). 'Do you want to do some arm wrestling?' Children's strategies when experiencing domestic violence and the meaning of age. *Child & Family Social Work, 22*(2), 680–688. https://doi.org/10.1111/cfs.12283

Överlien, C., & Holt, S. (2018). Letter to the editor: Research on children experiencing domestic violence. *Journal of Family Violence, 34*(1), 65–67. https://doi.org/10.1007/s10896-018-9997-9

Överlien, C., & Hydén, M. (2009). Children's actions when experiencing domestic violence. *Childhood, 16*(4), 479–496. https://doi.org/10.1177/0907568209343757

Perry, B. D., Pollard, R. A., Blakley, T. L., Baker, W. L., & Vigilante, D. (1995). Childhood trauma, the neurobiology of adaptation, and "use-dependent" development of the brain: How "states" become "traits." *Infant Mental Health Journal, 16*(4), 271–291. https://doi.org/10.1002/1097-0355(199524)16:4<271::AID-IMHJ2280 160404>3.0.CO;2-B

Rose, N. (1985). *The psychological complex: Psychology, politics, and society in England, 1869–1939.* Routledge & Kegan Paul.

Rose, N. (2008). Psychology as a social science. *Subjectivity, 25*(1), 446–462. https://doi.org/10.1057/SUB.2008.30

Rose, N. (2010). 'Screen and intervene': Governing risky brains. *History of the Human Sciences, 23*(1), 79–105. https://doi.org/10.1177/0952695109352415

Rothschild, B. (2017). *The body remembers: Revolutionizing trauma treatment* (Vol. 2). W. W. Norton & Company.

Sokoloff, N. J., & Dupont, I. (2005). Domestic violence at the intersections of race, class, and gender. *Violence Against Women, 11*(1), 38–64. https://doi.org/10.1177/1077801204271476

Sousa, C., Herrenkohl, T. I., Moylan, C. A., Tajima, E. A., Klika, J. B., Herrenkohl, R. C., & Russo, M. J. (2011). Longitudinal study on the effects of child abuse and children's exposure to domestic violence, parent-child attachments, and antisocial behavior in adolescence. *Journal of Interpersonal Violence, 26*(1), 111–136. https://doi.org/10.1177/0886260510362883

Southwick, S. M., Bonanno, G. A., Masten, A. S., Panter-Brick, C., & Yehuda, R. (2014). Resilience definitions, theory, and challenges: Interdisciplinary perspectives. *European Journal of Psychotraumatology, 5*(1). https://doi.org/10.3402/ejpt.v5.25338

Suzuki, S. L., Geffner, R., & Bucky, S. F. (2008). The experiences of adults exposed to intimate partner violence as children: An exploratory qualitative study of resilience and protective factors. *Journal of Emotional Abuse*, 8(1–2), 103–121. https://doi.org/10.1080/10926790801984523

Swanston, J., Bowyer, L., & Vetere, A. (2014). Towards a richer understanding of school-age children's experiences of domestic violence: The voices of children and their mothers. *Clinical Child Psychology and Psychiatry*, 19(2), 184–201. https://doi.org/10.1177/1359104513485082

Thiara, R. K., & Humphreys, C. (2017). Absent presence: The ongoing impact of men's violence on the mother-child relationship. *Child & Family Social Work*, 22(1), 137–145. https://doi.org/10.1111/cfs.12210

Thomason, M. E., & Marusak, H. A. (2017). Toward understanding the impact of trauma on the early developing human brain. *Neuroscience*, 342, 55–67. https://doi.org/10.1016/J.NEUROSCIENCE.2016.02.022

UK Government. (2021). *Domestic Abuse Act 2021*. Domestic Abuse Act 2021. https://www.legislation.gov.uk/ukpga/2021/17/enacted

Uttal, W. (2011). *Mind and brain: A critical appraisal of cognitive neuroscience*. The MIT Press.

Valentine, G. (2003). Boundary crossings: transitions from childhood to adulthood. *Children's Geographies*, 1(1), 37–52. https://doi.org/10.1080/14733280302186

Walkerdine, V. (1993). Beyond Developmentalism? *Theory & Psychology*, 3(4), 451–469. https://doi.org/10.1177/0959354393034004

Wallace, S., Nazroo, J., & Bécares, L. (2016). Cumulative effect of racial discrimination on the mental health of ethnic minorities in the United Kingdom. *American Journal of Public Health*, 106(7), 1294–1300. https://doi.org/10.2105/AJPH.2016.303121

Wastell, D., & White, S. (2012). Blinded by neuroscience: Social policy, the family and the infant brain. *Families, Relationships and Societies*, 1(3), 397–414. https://doi.org/10.1332/204674312X656301

Zarse, E. M., Neff, M. R., Yoder, R., Hulvershorn, L., Chambers, J. E., & Chambers, R. A. (2019). The adverse childhood experiences questionnaire: Two decades of research on childhood trauma as a primary cause of adult mental illness, addiction, and medical diseases. *Cogent Medicine*, 6(1), 1581447. https://doi.org/10.1080/2331205X.2019.1581447

Zittoun, T. (2007). Symbolic resources and responsibility in transitions. *YOUNG*, 15(2), 193–211. https://doi.org/10.1177/110330880701500205

Zittoun, T. (2008). Learning through transitions: The role of institutions. *European Journal of Psychology of Education*, 23(2), 165–181. https://doi.org/10.1007/BF03172743

3
A FEMINIST PSYCHOLOGICAL PERSPECTIVE ON MEMORY, GENDER AND VOICE/S

Introduction

This chapter discusses how and why this book came to be about women's stories. It will explore the historical context that shapes how women's accounts and memories of violence have typically been considered uncredible or even false. I will consider the implications of this historical legacy in USA, European and UK contexts for how women are heard when they talk about violence and recall memories of childhood violence and abuse. This chapter explores why gender matters and then outlines how I understand feminism in the context of this work and what working with feminism as a life question might mean. This chapter goes on to outline the theoretical and philosophical underpinnings of my research with women and how I made sense of their accounts, highlighting why a focus on gender and voice/s was generative and an important way of embracing and doing feminism in this work.

Memory, historical legacies and why gender matters

When starting out on the work for this book, I did not initially set out to explore women's stories. However, when I was recruiting participants, it was only women who volunteered to participate. Therefore, this project became about women's accounts, and gender became an important part of how I understood their accounts. For this reason, it feels important to explore the historical context that shapes how women's accounts of abuse have historically been discredited and devalued and the implications of this history for how women tend to be heard when they talk about experiences of violence and abuse even now.

DOI: 10.4324/9781003393160-3

Traditionally, in psychology, memory has been studied by researchers and clinicians using quantitative experimental methods and hypothesis testing. Historically, at least in psychology, there has been an underpinning assumption that there is an objective reality relating to an event that should correlate with how a memory of such an event is stored and recalled. In other words, our experiences are, in a way, directly 'imprinted' into memory and are recalled, a bit like playing back a video of the event, in this directly imprinted and exact state. However, these laboratory and experimental conditions do not really replicate 'real-life', nor stressful, distressing, traumatic or even therapeutic conditions. As such, findings from these kinds of studies are not very applicable to real-life situations, particularly where there is violence or trauma or where a lot of time has passed. It is well recognised amongst contemporary cognitive, psychoanalytic, feminist and social constructionist clinicians and researchers who study memory that many factors shape processes of remembering, such as social context, environment, emotional state and new memories that have been stored since the original event took place (Otgaar et al., 2023). There is an understanding that memory is highly malleable, fluid and dynamic. And further, this 'over-objectifying' way of understanding the mind is too simplistic and not reflective of how humans interact within social, cultural and relational contexts (Campbell, 2003; Reavey & Brown, 2006). There is now an understanding that memory is a 'socially structured human activity' (Haaken & Reavey, 2010, p. 6) and that the truth of a memory can be seen as 'continually open to negotiation, questioning and reconstruction, depending on the context of its use' (Haaken & Reavey, 2010, p. 6).

We now have a theoretical and evidence-based understanding that 'our memory system is reconstructive, not reproductive' (Otgaar et al., 2023, p. 122). That memory and memory recall is a social, relational, fluid and dynamic process. However, there is a political history of memory shaped by patriarchal power structures, which shapes how women's memories of childhood violence are told and heard. In this section of the chapter, I discuss the legacy of what has historically been termed 'False Memory Syndrome'. That is, the belief that it is possible to recover childhood memories that are not true. The idea of 'False Memory Syndrome' first emerged in the early 1990s in the USA and UK media in response to adult survivors of childhood sexual abuse beginning to recall memories of the abuse and spoke out in public about their experiences in the 1980s. This was mainly in the USA, Canada, Europe and the UK, and it was at a time following the 1970s feminist movement, which opened spaces for women to speak more publicly about forms of violence such as domestic violence, sexual violence and incest. By the late 1980s, many women and some men were talking about childhood sexual abuse, which they did not have previous knowledge about, usually in therapy with the help of therapists who worked specifically with uncovering and addressing traumatic memories. These therapists were finding that symptoms such as depression and eating disorders were often a result of underlying and sometimes unremembered childhood abuse and these therapists felt it was morally wrong to disguise childhood sexual abuse with pathologising labels and treat these women as 'sick' when in fact their symptoms were a result of childhood sexual abuse that was kept concealed (Haaken & Reavey, 2010).

These 'recovered' memories resulted in a 'war' over memory, with academics, feminists, therapists and legal professionals debating whether these recovered memories were true or false (Campbell, 2003; Haaken & Reavey, 2010). Feminist-informed therapists and academics believed that believing women and validating their accounts was crucial. However, there was also a prevailing belief and outcry that these therapists could and did implant memories in the minds of women through talking in therapy, causing them to recover memories of childhood sexual abuse that were not true (Clancy et al., 2000; Williams & Banyard, 1999). There was a major backlash from those accused of perpetrating or enabling the sexual abuse ('wrongly accused' parents), arguing that these recovered memories were false (Brown & Burman, 1997). Discourses surrounding 'False Memory Syndrome' positioned therapists – mostly feminist-informed therapists and survivor activists – as destroying the lives of happy families because of recovered memories of abuse.

Academics on both sides of the memory 'war' began studying memory to try to understand what was happening with these recovered memories through therapy. It has been recognised now that much of the work in therapy, especially trauma therapy or therapy that addresses distressing childhood experiences, is to address and re-story the past. As such, this can be a form of remembering, examining how memories might have been assigned meanings over time and how life experiences might shape memories of past events and broader social-cultural worlds (Haaken & Reavey, 2010).

What stands out is that an anti-feminist rhetoric weaves through these debates about whether these reclaimed memories were true or false. Some even claimed that these feminist therapists were, in fact, anti-feminist because by recovering previously forgotten memories, they were turning otherwise happy and healthy women into patients in a system that was set up to pathologise them. The fact that disclosures led to women being institutionalised in psychiatric systems that were set up to pathologise has also been argued from within feminist psychology too (Kitzinger & Perkins, 1993). This points towards the difficulty of women's stories of violence being taken seriously in a context where they then risk their difficulties relating to trauma and abuse becoming diagnosed, medicalised and pathologised through therapeutic and psychiatric discourses and systems of power where professionals occupy positions of status and power over their clients/patients. Some have also argued that this debate about whether the memories were true or false was, more broadly, a symptom of Western cultural trends (Schuman &

Galvez, 1996), including the cultural crisis in Western post-1970s feminism and women's liberation around gender, sexuality and authority (Haaken & Reavey, 2010). *Something* was happening here, regardless of what was 'true', where women in their masses were coming forward with disclosures of childhood distress and violence, and there was a social 'hysteria' and moral outcry about whether what they were saying was true.

This is an issue of gender, politics and epistemic justice. This cultural and historical context in the USA, Canada and Europe/UK contributed to a discourse of 'dis-believability' of women's knowledge about experiences of violence and victimisation (Brown & Burman, 1997; Schuman & Galvez, 1996). While it could be argued that ideas surrounding 'False Memory Syndrome' are a thing of the past, they have a legacy that continues to shape the present. The notion of 'False Memory Syndrome' still threads through *why* women's accounts of abuse in childhood are so vulnerable to being discredited (Schuman & Galvez, 1996). For example, currently, if clients receiving therapy are about to give evidence in court about witnessing or experiencing abuse, then they must enter into what is called pre-trial therapy, whereby therapists are advised against discussing the event(s) directly, and are typically encouraged to use approaches which focus on day-to-day coping, feelings about the trial, and feelings about the event(s) rather than details of the event(s), in case the therapy somehow interferes with memory (Fouché & Fouché, 2017; Pace, 2001). This book is not about childhood sexual abuse, and it does not ask questions about the accuracy, truth or falsehood of memory. However, these discourses about the dis-believability and untrustworthiness of women's memories of abuse in childhood are important to consider as they provide powerful narrative frameworks and historical and political context for how and why women tell their stories and how they are heard.

Remembering and talking about violence: 'truth' and epistemic (in)justice

A range of psychological literature suggests that experiencing trauma can have a profound effect on memory and how we make meaning of our experiences and construct a sense of self. For example, when re-telling trauma memories, there can be a disconnect or rupture in narrative coherency and integration (Alcoff, 2018; Brison, 2002; Campbell, 2003; Herman, 2015). This means that there can be a rupture, a sense of disconnectedness or a struggle to integrate the 'before' and 'after', making it somewhat difficult to narrate a coherent and integrated sense of self or account of what has happened (Brison, 2002; Herman, 2015) that is perceived as legible or readable by others. As I write this book, I want to be cautious about the risk of pathologising stories that lack coherency due to the way that, historically, women's stories have been devalued. I want to be clear that I do not view narrative incoherency as a problem or a sign of deficit, a sign of personality 'disorder' or a sign of false memory.

Feminist scholars have argued that memory is as much about power and politics as it is about the event(s) that have occurred (Alcoff, 2018). Gender matters here because issues of truth, reliability and accuracy of the account are routinely called into question when women talk about violence or abuse that has happened to them in their lives. As I have explored above, the notion of recovering memories that are not true is located in patriarchal power structures whereby the 'myth of objectivity' (Brown & Burman, 1997, p. 10) is pervasive in society, in psychiatric systems and in therapeutic and legal contexts. Women's stories of abuse have tended to be treated with caution, from the starting point that they may not be believable and that an objective version of reality exists and should be counted as 'truth' (Alcoff, 2012; Woodiwiss, 2007, 2014). This is despite contemporary research and understandings of memory, which tell us this is not how memory works. With this in mind, I intentionally centre gendered power structures in this book, recognising, as Woodiwiss et al. (2017) highlighted, that there is a 'history to women's storytelling that has seen women or aspects of women's lives repeatedly removed or silenced…' (p. 16). Such epistemic privileging needs to be critically examined. In the context of childhood domestic violence, for people whose childhoods were characterised by coercion and violence, their voices and accounts of these experiences are likely to have already been silenced through power structures that view children as vulnerable, unable to speak or lacking credibility when they do.

Getting underneath what we mean by 'truth' matters. As noted by Motzkau and Jefferson (2009), critical approaches in psychology take seriously the role that methods have in challenging mainstream and dominant assumptions and, as such, challenging what is held up as 'true'. The assumptions that underpin how we come to know what we know – referred to as epistemic practices – are as important to examine as the methods we use to generate data. Typically, in psychology and related professions, values of empiricism and objectivity have dominated. Empiricism refers to the privileging of information that can be measured, controlled and separated from emotion – 'objective' knowledge – and an undervaluing of lived-experience-based, observable 'subjective' knowledge. As such, not all evidence is counted as equal (Hunsley & Mash, 2007), and there is an evidence hierarchy that determines the theories and practices we use and what is held as 'true' (Ghaemi, 2010).

The implications of these 'truths' are vast for all of us: researchers, practitioners, those of us with personal lived experience and those of us – like myself – who occupy multiple positions. This is one of the reasons why I am drawn to feminist research. Feminist research exposes the ways in which intersectional systems of marginalisation, oppression and power are upheld by conclusions derived from psychological 'science'. As such, feminist research holds that it is crucial to examine power relations in any process of knowledge production (Wigginton & Lafrance, 2019). This is particularly relevant in the context of domestic violence research and work, where power is a central part of how domestic violence is perpetrated, maintained and experienced, *and* it is a central part of how 'truths' about domestic violence become known.

Epistemic justice has been defined as 'a harm done to a person in her capacity as an epistemic subject (a knower, a reasoner, a questioner) by undermining her capacity to engage in epistemic practices such as giving knowledge to others (testifying) or making sense of one's experiences (interpreting). It typically arises when a hearer does not take the statements of a speaker as seriously as they deserve to be taken' (Crichton et al., 2017, p. 65). Miranda Fricker has written extensively about epistemic injustice, and I draw on her definitions and distinctions here to orient this book to this concept. She proposes that there are two main kinds of epistemic injustice: testimonial injustice and hermeneutical injustice. She describes testimonial injustice as an issue primarily about prejudice. She defines it as 'if prejudice on the hearer's part causes him to give less credibility to the speaker than he would otherwise have given' (Fricker, 2007, p. 4). She locates testimonial injustice as related to broader patterns and systems of social injustice, acknowledging that prejudice can be in the form of identity prejudice (e.g. a Black woman may be less likely to be believed by the police because of racism). Hermeneutical injustice is about a gap in hermeneutic resources between speaker and listener or between social groups. Fricker defines hermeneutical injustice as being when a person 'cannot properly comprehend her own experience, let alone render it communicatively intelligible to others. I explain this sort of epistemic injustice as stemming from a gap in collective hermeneutical resources – a gap, that is, in our shared tools of social interpretation – where it is no accident that the cognitive disadvantage created by this gap impinges unequally on different social groups' (Fricker, 2007, p. 6). For example, this might be a person explaining an experience of coercive control, before coercive control was a known and more widely accepted concept. Fricker considers both forms of epistemic injustice as located in broader systems of power, privilege and oppression.

To return to the issue of childhood domestic violence, young women's accounts, and why epistemic justice matters, as I discussed in Chapter 2, a small amount of qualitative research spanning the last couple of decades has explored the experiences of adults who experienced domestic violence as children (for example, Anderson & Danis, 2006; Gonzales et al., 2012; Humphreys, 2001; O'Brien et al., 2013; Suzuki et al., 2008). This research points to the importance of centring lived experiences with the more recently published studies I discussed advocating for the importance of attending to context, power and gender in terms of how adults are impacted by childhood domestic violence and how they make sense of their experiences. However, biologising and individualising assumptions about development, resilience and distress are evident even in current research, which appears to privilege outcome-based essentialising approaches that leave an overarching message that exposure to violence leaves lasting damage by interfering with and disrupting 'normal' brain development (Thomason & Marusak, 2017). I discussed that underpinning this 'resilient brain' discourse (Burman, 2017) is a dominant biomedical and scientific understanding of distress, resilience and identity. These underpinning assumptions do not make space for alternative narratives to be told or heard. As feminist psychologists have argued, this biomedical discourse dominates as it has the capacity and power to construct a particular version of 'truth' and reality that is bolstered and upheld by the economic, political and institutional power of medicine and science (Lafrance & McKenzie-Mohr, 2013). This dominance of psy-discourses that are presented as scientific truths (Marecek & Lafrance, 2021) provides limiting and limited knowledge about children's trajectories to adulthood after domestic violence, importantly, obscuring the multiplicity of lived experience voices. The impacts and outcomes of childhood domestic violence are not always predictable in adulthood, and these theoretical perspectives have not sufficiently paid attention to how individuals make sense of their present-day selves and relationships through the lens of their childhood experiences. My hope is that this book takes up a feminist lens to address some of these issues.

Working with feminism as a life question

With the above in mind, I want to outline how I come to think of feminism and embody feminism, particularly in the context of this book. Drawing on the writings of Sara Ahmed (2017), I understand feminism as a life question that guides how I try to live out my life and how I aim to conduct my work. In this section of the chapter, I outline how I conceptualise feminist thinking and use it to guide my thinking about this work. It is far beyond the scope of this book to fully engage with the history of feminisms and critically examine where we find ourselves in the current landscape of domestic violence work and feminist thinking. However, it is important to acknowledge that feminism is not a single theory, and there is no single political goal or strategy (Rupp & Taylor, 1999). Diverse ideas about feminist thought and feminist politics and theory exist, and feminisms are in many ways situated in social, cultural and political contexts. As Macleod et al. (2014) have noted, 'every feminism bears the stamp of the material conditions, ideological presuppositions and socio-political structures of its place of origin' (p. 6). Critiques of 'Western feminisms' argue that 'feminism' as situated in Western, European and USA contexts only speaks to a minority elite group of women and, as such, does not centre the interests of, or experiences of, the majority of the global female population. This localisation of feminisms is important to acknowledge and has historically remained largely unaddressed within Europe and the USA (Kurian, 2001).

Broadly speaking, in the UK-based European context that I am in, feminist psychologists have an interest in examining individual experiences within their socio-cultural contexts, and they are specifically interested in gender inequalities and the marginalisation and oppression of women in a patriarchal (Western) context. There is an interest in the systems that enable patriarchal and oppressive power relations to continue in old and new ways. I note the cultural and local specificity of feminisms because, of course, I, myself, am located within a culture that conceptualises and 'does' feminisms in particular Eurocentric and Westernised ways. In doing this work, I hope some of my work does something to critically examine systems of power, privilege and oppression that uphold epistemic practices, ways of knowing and ways of listening.

Drawing on Sara Ahmed's extensive thinking and writing on feminist thought (Ahmed, 2014, 2017), she has argued that feminism is work that extends beyond what one considers as traditional 'work' and it seeps into most aspects of our being. As such, she argues that feminism is what we live, and it is a way of living in this world, a set of values and beliefs that orient us towards a way of being. I would argue that feminism is understood and lived out differently according to each of our unique histories, values and beliefs. To me, this means living and working in a way that values justice, seeks to address inequalities and harm and takes seriously the intersectional aspects of privilege and marginalisation, and how these operate at micro and macro levels personally, locally and globally. It is not only a mind-based activity of theorising that which we encounter or read. It is an embodied way of being and relating to all forms of human and non-human life. I am most drawn to Sara Ahmed's understandings of feminism, as she writes about making feminism a life question, and living out feminism in how we live our lives. She has written that living feminism out means 'asking ethical questions about how to live better in an unjust and unequal world... how to create relationships with others that are more equal; how to find ways to support those who are not supported or are less supported by social systems; how to keep coming up against histories that have become concrete, histories that have become as solid as walls' (Ahmed, 2017, p. 1). What also resonates well with me and my thinking is how Ahmed writes about the diverse ways we might have of refusing and rebelling against that which has harmed us. She wrote that the word feminism 'brings to mind loud acts of refusal and rebellion as well as the quiet ways we might have of not holding onto things that diminish us' (Ahmed, 2017, p. 1).

These understandings of feminist thinking guide my work in this book. I hope that the following chapters reflect critical, relational, reflexive and attentive bodymind work. I discuss the idea of bodymind work more in Chapter 8, but in summary, it refers to a way of being and working that extends beyond the cognitive and intellectual task of theorising. It is embodied, expansive and generative, inclusive of mind and body, rather than body and mind as separable. For clarity and ease of reading, I have summarised my sense of how I understand feminism in the following six guiding principles that I view as central to violence research that seeks to address power and epistemic injustice.

1 Valuing relationality and dialogue. This includes valuing all human and non-human lifeforms and rejecting human-centric, oppressive and patriarchal hierarchical ways of viewing what and whose life and voice matters.
2 Working to address and examine systems that uphold epistemic and social injustices.
3 Understanding that personal lived experiences are political.
4 Understanding that it is crucial to examine power relations in any process of knowledge production (Harding, 1990). This means critically examining colonial ways of thinking that uphold knowledge hierarchies, which keep particular kinds of knowledge centred and actively marginalises and discredits knowledges that do not align with the status quo.
5 Embracing bodymind ways of thinking and being that view selfhood as plural and embodied. This means valuing and crediting knowledge rooted in embodied ways of knowing.
6 Embracing 'voice' as plural.

In the spirit of feminism being a life question, feminism is directly and inextricably related to questions of knowledge, truth and reality. So, epistemological and ontological questions such as 'What kind of knowledge counts?' and 'Do I believe there to be one globally shared version of reality, or can I understand there are multiple versions of and experiences of reality, and all hold legitimacy and validity?' deeply guide how we work with and consider the credibility and value of stories that are shared with us. As I will go on to explore in this chapter, gender matters when listening to stories of violence, and when understanding how people talk about violence. Women, especially when talking about violence or trauma, are not held up as authoritative knowledge producers, particularly if their stories are told in ways that change over time or do not align with what it might be expected they 'should' say (Alcoff, 1991; Woodiwiss, 2014) or if they already experience identity-based prejudice. Feminist qualitative research has typically sought to challenge the myth of objective knowledge production and the marginalisation of women's voices by centralising women's voices and viewing women as offering valuable knowledge about their own lives (Doucet & Mauthner, 2008; hooks, 1990; Kitzinger & Perkins, 1993; Woodiwiss et al., 2017).

I position this work within a relational and dialogical way of thinking about how knowledge is produced (epistemology) and about what reality is (ontology). In line with this, I draw on Haraway's (1988) feminist politics of knowledge production (also see Hinton, 2014; Mauthner & Doucet, 2003; Nencel, 2014; Wilkinson & Kitzinger, 2013). This is an assumption that knowledges and realities are situated, located and produced relationally (Mauthner & Doucet, 2003). It is an assumption that multiple realities exist and that they are constructed through interactions with others, and in relation to social and cultural contexts (Haraway, 1988). As such, my approach in this work is that I embrace and value individual stories and subjectivities, *and* I am interested in examining how the contexts in which they are told shape *how* they are told. From this view, knowledge is always situated. Feminist research advocates the value of plural philosophies because it enables attention to how subjectivities and personal stories are intertwined with and situated in social, cultural and political contexts (Thompson et al., 2018; Yuval-Davis, 2006).

Summary

In this chapter, I have discussed the historical and political contexts that shape epistemic practices when listening to women's experiences of childhood violence and abuse. I have briefly outlined the history of the idea of 'False Memory Syndrome' in USA, Canada, European and UK contexts where women's discoveries of memories of childhood sexual abuse in the 1970s and 1980s were part of what some have deemed a social 'hysteria' and 'memory wars' where clinicians, researchers, families and activists sought to determine whether uncovered memories were true or false. Patriarchal structures are organised in a way that privileges objectivity and stability – that is, unchanging memories that are seen as direct representations of events. This means that women's accounts of violence and abuse in childhood are more likely to be discredited, and women are more likely to be treated with the premise that they may not be believable or trustworthy sources of knowledge.

Even though this study is not concerned with assessing truth and falsehood, examining how women's narratives have historically been devalued is necessary. As Paula Nicholson has noted, the study of domestic violence and abuse is a complex process and 'needs to take account of history and culture, gender-power relations and the material context, as well as the changing dynamics of emotion and psychology' (Nicholson, 2019, p. 6). Considered in this way, gender matters when we think about memory and remembering childhood violence. Attending to gendered histories and socio-cultural contexts is part of a feminist way of working and is considered an important listening method. I have discussed that in this book, unstable storylines and narrative instability are not considered indicators of an unreliable narrator; rather, these are products of how we talk and how the self is constructed. It is these sites of instability and multivocality that are precisely of interest in the chapters that follow in this book. Lastly, this chapter has outlined what it means to take a feminist approach in this work, and I have described that feminism in the context of this work is a life question guided by an aim to attend to power and address epistemic injustices. I consider that to do this, relationships, embodiment and embracing 'voice' as plural are crucial commitments to me. I highlight 'to me' to recognise that 'feminisms' is a plural concept, and we each may approach doing feminism and being feminist in unique ways. In the following chapter, I turn attention to how I did the research that this book is about, and I come back to these understandings of feminist work, feminist questions and epistemic practices.

References

Ahmed, S. (2014). *The cultural politics of emotion* (2nd ed.). Edinburgh University Press.
Ahmed, S. (2017). *Living a feminist life*. Duke University Press.
Alcoff, L. (1991). The problem of speaking for others. *Cultural Critique, 20*, 5–32. https://doi.org/10.2307/1354221
Alcoff, L. (2012). Feminism: Then and now. *The Journal of Speculative Philosophy, 26*(2), 268–290. https://doi.org/10.5325/jspecphil.26.2.0268
Alcoff, L. (2018). *Rape and resistance*. Polity Press.
Anderson, K. M., & Danis, F. S. (2006). Adult daughters of battered women: Resistance and resilience in the face of danger. *Affilia, 21*(4), 419–432. https://doi.org/10.1177/0886109906292130
Brison, S. (2002). *Aftermath: Violence and the remaking of a self*. Princeton University Press.
Brown, L. S., & Burman, E. (1997). Feminist responses to the 'false memory' debate. *Feminism & Psychology, 7*(1), 7–16. https://doi.org/10.1177/0959353597071002
Burman, E. (2017). *Deconstructing developmental psychology* (3rd ed.). Routledge.
Campbell, S. (2003). *Relational remembering: Rethinking the memory wars*. Rowman & Littlefield Publishers.
Clancy, S. A., Schacter, D. L., McNally, R. J., & Pitman, R. K. (2000). False recognition in women reporting recovered memories of sexual abuse. *Psychological Science, 11*(1), 26–31. https://doi.org/10.1111/1467-9280.00210
Crichton, P., Carel, H., & Kidd, I. J. (2017). Epistemic injustice in psychiatry. *BJPsych Bulletin, 41*(2), 65–70. https://doi.org/10.1192/PB.BP.115.050682
Doucet, A., & Mauthner, N. S. (2008). What can be known and how? Narrated subjects and the Listening Guide. *Qualitative Research, 8*(3), 399–409. https://doi.org/10.1177/1468794106093636
Fouché, A., & Fouché, D. F. (2017). Pre-trial therapy for child witnesses in cases of sexual abuse: A scoping literature review. *Journal of Psychology in Africa, 27*(5), 462–471. https://doi.org/10.1080/14330237.2017.1375201
Fricker, M. (2007). *Epistemic injustice: Power and the ethics of knowing*. Oxford University Press.
Ghaemi, S. N. (2010). Levels of evidence. *Psychiatric Times, 27*(1), 1–4.
Gonzales, G., Chronister, K. M., Linville, D., & Knoble, N. B. (2012). Experiencing parental violence: A qualitative examination of adult men's resilience. *Psychology of Violence, 2*(1), 90–103. https://doi.org/10.1037/a0026372
Haaken, J., & Reavey, P. (2010). Why memory still matters. Disturbing recollections. In J. Haaken & P. Reavey (Eds.), *Memory matters: Contexts for understanding sexual abuse recollections*. Routledge.
Haraway, D. (1988). Situated knowledges: The science question in feminism and the privilege of partial perspective. *Feminist Studies, 14*(3), 575. https://doi.org/10.2307/3178066

Harding, S. (1990). Feminism and theories of scientific knowledge. *Women: A Cultural Review*, 1(1), 87–98. https://doi.org/10.1080/09574049008578026

Herman, J. (2015). *Trauma and recovery*. Basic Books.

Hinton, P. (2014). 'Situated knowledges' and new materialism(s): Rethinking a politics of location. *Women: A Cultural Review*, 25(1), 99–113. https://doi.org/10.1080/09574042.2014.901104

hooks, b. (1990). *Yearning: Race, gender, and cultural politics*. South End Press.

Humphreys, C. (2001). Growing up in a violent home: The lived experience of daughters of battered women. *Journal of Family Nursing*, 7(3), 244–260. https://doi.org/10.1177/107484070100700303

Hunsley, J., & Mash, E. J. (2007). Evidence-based assessment. *Annual Review of Clinical Psychology*, 3, 29–51. https://doi.org/10.1146/annurev.clinpsy.3.022806.091419

Kitzinger, C., & Perkins, R. (1993). *Changing our minds: Lesbian feminism and psychology*. New York University Press.

Kurian, A. (2001). Feminism and the developing world. In S. Gamble (Ed.), *The Routledge companion to feminism and postfeminism* (2nd ed.). Routledge.

Lafrance, M. N., & McKenzie-Mohr, S. (2013). The DSM and its lure of legitimacy. *Feminism & Psychology*, 23(1), 119–140. https://doi.org/10.1177/0959353512467974

Macleod, C., Marecek, J., & Capdevila, R. (2014). Feminism & psychology going forward. *Feminism & Psychology*, 24(1), 3–17. https://doi.org/10.1177/0959353513515308

Marecek, J., & Lafrance, M. N. (2021). Editorial introduction: The politics of psychological suffering. *Feminism & Psychology*, 31(1), 3–18. https://doi.org/10.1177/0959353521989537

Mauthner, N. S., & Doucet, A. (2003). Reflexive accounts and accounts of reflexivity in qualitative data analysis. *Sociology*, 37(3), 413–431. https://doi.org/10.1177/00380385030373002

Motzkau, J. F., & Jefferson, A. M. (2009). Editorial: Research as practice: On critical methodologies 1. *Qualitative Research in Psychology*, 6(1–2), 1–11. https://doi.org/10.1080/14780880902896416

Nencel, L. (2014). Situating reflexivity: Voices, positionalities and representations in feminist ethnographic texts. *Women's Studies International Forum*, 43, 75–83. https://doi.org/10.1016/j.wsif.2013.07.018

Nicholson, P. (2019). *Domestic violence and psychology. Critical perspectives on intimate partner violence and abuse* (2nd ed.). Routledge.

O'Brien, K. L., Cohen, L., Pooley, J. A., & Taylor, M. F. (2013). Lifting the domestic violence cloak of silence: Resilient Australian women's reflected memories of their childhood experiences of witnessing domestic violence. *Journal of Family Violence*, 28(1), 95–108. https://doi.org/10.1007/s10896-012-9484-7

Otgaar, H., Dodier, O., Garry, M., Howe, M. L., Loftus, E. F., Lynn, S. J., Mangiulli, I., McNally, R. J., & Patihis, L. (2023). Oversimplifications and misrepresentations in the repressed memory debate: A reply to Ross. *Journal of Child Sexual Abuse*, 32(1), 116–126. https://doi.org/10.1080/10538712.2022.2133043

Pace, M. (2001). Therapy for child witnesses prior to a criminal trial; training implications. *Child Abuse Review*, 10(4), 279–285. https://doi.org/10.1002/car.698

Reavey, P., & Brown, S. D. (2006). Transforming past agency and action in the present. *Theory & Psychology*, 16(2), 179–202. https://doi.org/10.1177/0959354306062535

Rupp, L. J., & Taylor, V. (1999). Forging feminist identity in an international movement: A collective identity approach to twentieth-century feminism. *Signs: Journal of Women in Culture and Society, 24*(2), 362–386. https://doi.org/10.1086/495344

Schuman, J., & Galvez, M. (1996). A meta/multi-discursive reading of 'false memory syndrome'. *Feminism & Psychology, 6*(1), 7–29. https://doi.org/10.1177/0959353596061002

Suzuki, S. L., Geffner, R., & Bucky, S. F. (2008). The experiences of adults exposed to intimate partner violence as children: An exploratory qualitative study of resilience and protective factors. *Journal of Emotional Abuse, 8*(1–2), 103–121. https://doi.org/10.1080/10926790801984523

Thomason, M. E., & Marusak, H. A. (2017). Toward understanding the impact of trauma on the early developing human brain. *Neuroscience, 342*, 55–67. https://doi.org/10.1016/J.NEUROSCIENCE.2016.02.022

Thompson, L., Rickett, B., & Day, K. (2018). Feminist relational discourse analysis: Putting the personal in the political in feminist research. *Qualitative Research in Psychology, 15*(1), 93–115. https://doi.org/10.1080/14780887.2017.1393586

Wigginton, B., & Lafrance, M. N. (2019). Learning critical feminist research: A brief introduction to feminist epistemologies and methodologies. *Feminism & Psychology, 0*(0), 1–17. https://doi.org/10.1177/0959353519866058

Wilkinson, S., & Kitzinger, C. (2013). Representing our own experience: Issues in "insider" research. *Psychology of Women Quarterly, 37*(2), 251–255. https://doi.org/10.1177/0361684313483111

Williams, L. M., & Banyard, V. L. (1999). *Trauma and memory*. SAGE Publications.

Woodiwiss, J. (2007). Politics, responsibility and adult victims of childhood sexual abuse. *Sociological Research Online, 12*(2), 1–12. https://doi.org/10.5153/sro.1404

Woodiwiss, J. (2014). Beyond a single story: The importance of separating 'harm' from 'wrongfulness' and 'sexual innocence' from 'childhood' in contemporary narratives of childhood sexual abuse. *Sexualities, 17*(1–2), 139–158. https://doi.org/10.1177/1363460713511104

Woodiwiss, J., Smith, K., & Lockwood, K. (2017). *Feminist narrative research: Opportunities and challenges*. Palgrave Macmillan UK.

Yuval-Davis, N. (2006). Intersectionality and feminist politics. *European Journal of Women's Studies, 13*(3), 193–209. https://doi.org/10.1177/1350506806065752

4
INTERVIEWING WOMEN AND WORKING WITH POEMS

Introduction

This chapter outlines what drew me to narrative as a research methodology. I describe how I conducted the interviews with the research participants, who the participants were and how I used a feminist dialogical approach to listen to and make sense of women's stories. This chapter also briefly discusses the feminist ontological and epistemological underpinnings of my research and why these philosophical underpinnings were particularly necessary for listening to and working with young women's accounts of domestic violence.

A note about the terms 'narrative' and 'stories'

I use the terms 'narrative' and 'stories', and I want to take a moment to explain what they mean in the context of this book. In its most basic form, storytelling is what we do when we communicate something about ourselves or something about things that have happened in our lives. As such, 'stories' are defined as what people say about events or experiences. Importantly, I understand stories as having 'multiplicities of meanings' (Tamboukou, 2008, p. 283), and as such, there is no singular 'truth' but multiple. Epistemologically, my research was grounded in an understanding that knowledge is situated and co-constructed relationally and dialogically. As such, I view stories as neither static direct accounts of lived experience nor as accounts told only through socially and culturally grounded discourses (Andrews et al., 2013).

Perhaps in contradiction to how stories are typically understood, stories in this book are not viewed as coherent linear narratives. They may not have a beginning, middle and end, and they may never be finalised or complete

DOI: 10.4324/9781003393160-4

(Hermans, 2003). In my research, I was not interested in examining the structure or sequence of stories, although this is a valid approach to narrative analysis. Instead, I was interested in what kinds of stories were told and how they were told. It should be noted that 'stories' should not be confused with the notion of storytelling as fantasy, made-up or for fun or leisure.

'Narratives', on the other hand, are different to 'stories'. 'Narratives' refers to the resources people draw on to tell their stories. So, the stories we tell are shaped by narrative resources. The narrative resources we draw on when we tell stories are understood as shaped by the power relations at play in particular times, places and spaces (Andrews et al., 2013; Hermans, 2008). The assumption is that when people tell stories, they draw on the particular social, cultural or political narrative resources that are available to them at that time. A narrative resource refers to a set of meanings, dominant ideologies or understandings that exist within social and cultural spheres (Livholts & Tamboukou, 2015; Taylor, 2010). Arthur Frank, whose work centres around illness, ethics and narrative, primarily informed by sociological thinking, has explained this as our 'sense of selfhood is constructed and constrained by the resources we have available to tell our own story, as well as by the stories that are told about people like us' (Frank, 2012, p. 4). In my research, I was interested in what kinds of narrative resources shaped young women's accounts of domestic violence in childhood.

The research

One of the things I held as a key importance throughout this research was an epistemological commitment to value lived experience as a legitimate, valid and meaningful source of knowledge. I knew it was important that I spoke with young women directly about their stories, and that I listened carefully to what they had to say. Lived experience as a source of knowledge is not new to social science research (Andrews et al., 2013; Hollway & Jefferson, 2000; Mishler, 1986). However, it is particularly important in feminist research where listening to storied accounts from women is, in some ways, a resistance to knowledge hierarchies. Knowledge hierarchies in psychology refer to mainstream psychology's tendency to value knowledge produced through objective, patriarchal and colonised lenses and a devaluing of subjective forms of knowledge, knowledge coming from marginalised voices (Grzanka, 2018; Harel-Shalev & Daphna-Tekoah, 2021), or knowledge that offers truths that diverge from the norm or status quo.

Recruiting participants

I used social media (Twitter, now known as X) to share a call for participants. I should note, this was before Elon Musk bought and took over ownership of Twitter/X, and I no longer use this platform. I did, however, use the social media platform to connect with and reach people far beyond my personal connections. For this reason, it felt like a good space to reach people and organisations I might not know personally, but who were likely to have some interests or connections similar to mine. The call for participants explained that I was interested in speaking with young adults who had experienced domestic violence in childhood, lived in the UK, had not accessed any form of formal domestic abuse support in childhood and felt willing to speak about their experiences in an interview with me. I hoped social media would enable participants to contact me in ways that felt safe and comfortable to them. I recruited participants over a period of 12 months between July 2017 and July 2018. I posted on Twitter several times during these 12 months. My experience of recruitment was slow, but it was steady. The tweet advertising the study and inviting people to contact me was shared by accounts from a range of people, including individuals (academics, practitioners and people with a range of backgrounds) and organisations (some of these were organisations in the domestic abuse, sexual violence or violence against women area).

I was particularly interested in talking with people who had not accessed formal domestic abuse support as a child. This is because, as discussed in Chapter 1, I found that most of the existing research was based on the experiences of people who had been recruited through domestic abuse services. I then learnt that, given that most children do not access these services, existing knowledge was based only on the experiences of a minority of people, and there was a large group of people whose experiences were excluded from research. Based on my own experiences of interviewing children who were accessing services, I also felt that the specific context of accessing a service shaped their stories and *how* they told their stories to me.

As discussed in Chapter 2, domestic abuse services are variable across different locations in England due to the commissioning of services, the allocation of resources and variable risk assessment and needs assessment thresholds, which children and families may have to meet in order to have a service made available to them. Also, it was highly likely that due to the different timeframes and the range of ages that participants were during the domestic violence, the services that may have been available at the time would have varied greatly. For these reasons, I did not state what kind of support or service specifically, but when recruiting participants, I highlighted that I was interested in the experiences of those who did not receive formal support to address their experiences of domestic violence.

The participants

Relying on social media meant 'going with' the participants who volunteered. It became evident that more than ten participants would not be necessary because of the depth of interview content and the layers of analysis required. Due to the flexibility offered by narrative methodologies, there is a range of ways of doing narrative analysis, and there is no guide for how many participants should be recruited (Andrews et al., 2013). From looking at published studies using narrative analysis, I found significant variance in sample sizes ranging from 1 to around 50. I stopped recruitment once ten participants had been interviewed. I felt a larger sample size would not allow for the required attention to complexity and nuance without losing the context of the individual stories. Additionally, within a narrative and qualitative paradigm, additional participants would likely not add any more weight to the study conclusions, as there is not an interest in generalisability or uncovering a universal 'truth'; rather, the interest is in multiple situated 'truths' (Andrews et al., 2013; Riessman, 2008).

In the end, ten young women participated in interviews that were held between August 2017 and August 2018. Although the inclusion criteria did not specify gender, all participants were women. The women I interviewed all have experiences that can be considered as relatively excluded from existing dominant literature and as not neatly fitting into a singular category. These experiences include the fact they had not accessed specialist domestic abuse support. Further context about participants' lives is detailed – and I have taken care to anonymise details that might make them identifiable – in Table 4.1. It also feels pertinent to outline some of the ways that women I spoke with brought histories and life experiences with them that meant they diverged from normative expectations and that evidence domestic violence was far from the only concern that shaped their experiences. For example, four participants spoke about experiencing significant mental health difficulties, two had experienced multiple forms of violence in addition to the domestic violence perpetrated by their fathers (child sexual exploitation and child sexual abuse), four participants experienced abuse towards themselves as well as parental domestic abuse, four participants had experienced the death of a parent or sibling, five had grown up with their parent using violence or abuse towards multiple partners and eight participants specifically spoke about their parents' struggles with alcohol, mental ill-health or disabilities that they felt shaped their childhoods significantly and three were carers for a member of their family. It feels important to highlight these because these kinds of experiences do not neatly fit into one single category of 'exposure' to childhood domestic violence, but rather, they represent a perhaps more realistic picture of the lives children and young adults lead during and after childhood domestic violence.

Participants lived in a range of rural and urban locations in England. They are women who are students, professionals, those with academic or professional interest in psychology or domestic abuse and those who did not talk about an interest in these subjects. They come from a range of socioeconomic backgrounds and family contexts. However, it is important to note that the women I spoke with were a fairly educated group, as all but two were educated to degree level and some were studying at postgraduate level or had experience working in the domestic abuse field. However, one participant spoke extensively about her experience that her professional role in the domestic violence field had at many times prevented her from feeling able to voice the struggles of her childhood. The domestic abuse women I spoke to had experienced includes physical, emotional, sexual, psychological and financial. As I outlined above, when participants provided accounts of their childhoods and recoveries, these accounts were not about domestic abuse in isolation but mostly where domestic abuse intersects with other kinds of violence, challenges or 'otherness' that shaped their lives.

Participant details are provided in Table 4.1, based on what participants described in interviews. At the time of the research, I felt I wanted to respect participants' right to anonymity and make the interview process as least invasive as I could. Therefore, I did not formally collect demographic information from participants. In retrospect, this is something I would do differently, as collecting this information would enable a more intersectionality-informed analysis. However, interviews were in-depth, and participants did share aspects of their identities and experiences that provided some socio-cultural and identity-based information about who they were and their histories. In some ways, my guess is that they shared these parts of themselves where they felt able to, where they felt comfortable to, or where it felt relevant to or connected to the part of their story they were narrating. Even in writing the book now, I still feel that this felt the least-invasive way of gathering information about women who participated. At the time, I wanted to take as many measures as possible to try to re-distribute power in the interview and honour the storytelling agency of women, including how and when they disclosed or shared parts of who they were. Where I can, I include this identity and demographic information in the table below. However, because I did not formally and systematically collect this data, there are obvious gaps. Participant information is anonymised, and I have used pseudonyms. Participants were aged between 21 and 35. I have not included their ages here, and I have changed some identifiable information, to respect their anonymity.

The interviews

Before the interviews, I met the participant or had a conversation on the phone about what participation would involve, checking eligibility to participate and addressing any questions. After providing informed consent, interviews took place in various locations, including participants' homes, university rooms or on Skype or the phone (as chosen by each participant). Interviews lasted between 75 minutes and 135 minutes (average length: 91 minutes).

TABLE 4.1

Participant	Summary of information about the participant
Frances	Frances was a university student, and we conducted an in-person interview. The domestic violence she experienced was between her mother and father, and she described both parents as abusive. She also experienced direct abuse herself throughout most of her childhood from both parents (physical, emotional and psychological). During the interview, Frances also discussed experiences of mental illness, specifically experiencing an eating disorder, and the death of a sibling.
Clara	Clara was a university student, and we did an in-person interview. The domestic violence she experienced was her father's violence (physical, psychological and financial) towards her mother. In the interview, she emphasised the financial and emotional abuse that she recalled, and the ways in which she felt her father still controlled several aspects of her life. Clara also had caring responsibilities for her sibling who had significant learning disability-related needs.
Sonia	The interview with Sonia was on the phone. Sonia's sense was that a phone interview allowed her to speak more freely and granted her further layers of anonymity which she felt more comfortable with. The domestic violence she experienced was her father's violence against her mother, including physical and emotional abuse. She described that her mother was also abusive by re-directing her father's violence and abuse towards herself and her siblings. Sonia also discussed experiences of an eating disorder when she was younger.
Bethany	The interview with Bethany was on the phone. Bethany was a postgraduate student and was in employment too. Bethany felt that the phone granted her an additional layer of anonymity which enabled her to speak more freely. She described her childhood as constantly being around violence. The domestic violence she described was her father's on-going violence and abuse towards her mother. She described the domestic abuse as physical and emotional.
Liv	Liv was a university student. This interview was in-person. Liv's 'real dad' (her definition, referring to her biological father) was physically and emotionally abusive towards her mum. She also had an older brother who was violent when he was at home or when he would visit. Her biological father left when she was young, at which point her mother met a new partner whom Liv said then became the victim of her mother's violence. Liv had caring responsibilities for her mother who was disabled. She spoke about her suspected neurodivergence and experiences of mental illness and psychological distress relating to trauma.

(Continued)

Interviewing women and working with poems 47

TABLE 4.1 (Continued)

Participant	Summary of information about the participant
Emma	This interview was in-person. Emma was a postgraduate university student. She referred to growing up experiencing financial struggle, and she also referred to her neurodivergence during the interview. She discussed her experiences with mental ill-health, specifically anxiety. The domestic violence Emma experienced was her mother's abuse of her father. She described it as emotional, psychological and financial abuse. Emma took part in two in-person interviews.
Jasmine	Jasmine was a recent graduate and was in employment. The interview with Jasmine was via video call. The domestic violence that Jasmine experienced was her father's physical and emotional violence against her mother, and then her father's physical and emotional violence against his new female partner when he had left her mother. Jasmine visited her father and his partner over weekends. She experienced fear each time she visited and explained that she was too afraid to say to her mother she did not want to visit, but this had significant impacts on her over the years.
Nadine	The interview was in-person. Nadine was a university student who also discussed her neurodivergence and mental illnesses including eating disorders and PTSD. The domestic violence that Nadine experienced was her father's violence against her mother. She described the domestic abuse as extensive and severe, including sexual, physical, emotional and psychological violence. The abuse also included sexual and physical violence towards her.
Sochi	Sochi was a university student. This interview was face to face. The domestic violence that she experienced was not perpetrated by her biological father, but by her mother's several subsequent male partners after her biological father separated from her mother. She described the abuse as physical violence mostly. Sochi was the only visibly non-white participant (bearing in mind that two interviews were conducted via phone, and I did not ask participants about their race and ethnicity). She spoke about her racial identity and financial insecurity growing up at brief points during the interview.
Hayley	The interview with Hayley took place via Skype. During the interview, Hayley discussed her experiences with mental illness, relating to trauma and eating disorders. She also discussed growing up with financial insecurity. The domestic violence she experienced was physical violence from both parents (mother and father) towards each other. She did not name one as perpetrating the violence, but she described that sometimes her father directed the abuse towards her and her siblings instead of her mother.

I felt it was important to prioritise participants' choices by not assuming 'one size fits all' or that face-to-face interviews would suit everybody (Braun et al., 2017). I felt that offering options about their level of visibility and engagement (e.g. video, audio, face-to-face) was important, given that interviews would be about topics that could be considered sensitive. I wanted participants to feel as comfortable as possible. The value of choice about visibility was particularly notable for the participants who interviewed over the phone and explained that the anonymity of talking on the phone rather than video meant they felt more comfortable and at ease sharing in-depth personal experiences.

I approached the interviews with an interview guide that acted as a rough guide for myself and the participant on what topics we would likely discuss together. I shared the guide with participants in advance of the interviews. The interview guide is outlined in Box 4.1.

BOX 4.1   INTERVIEW GUIDE

Can you start by telling me a bit about yourself and your life experiences?
What was growing up like for you?
What were the things that helped you to cope with difficulties, including the domestic violence, when you were younger?
How do you feel about your childhood experiences now, and what sense do you make of those childhood experiences now?

Interviews were intentionally open and aimed to enable space for participants to structure their own telling of their stories. I used the interview guide flexibly, meaning interviews were a very open dialogue space that flowed organically. Narrative researchers advocate for using open, participant and story-led interviews, and are not structured by the interviewer only (Josselson, 2013; Riessman, 2008). I hoped that openness would enable participants to speak as freely as possible about things that they felt were relevant to their experiences. All interviews were audio-recorded with the participant's permission. To understand what the participants considered important aspects of their identity and lives and to learn more about their context, interviews started openly, and participants were invited to tell me a bit about themselves. This helped me get to know the participants and ease us both into the relational space.

I learnt a lot about interviewing in this open narrative style as I progressed through the year that I conducted the interviews. As I conducted interviews over a 12-month timeframe, I was able to transcribe and re-listen to interviews and begin analysis almost immediately after each interview had taken place. This meant that I could refine my listening practices and get more 'tuned in' to multivocality, where I noticed participants speaking from different voices. As such, I really valued the slow nature of interviewing and analysing during this year. I could refine my interviewing approach and learn to tune more into polyvocality in the moment in the interview and when listening to the recordings. Awareness in the moment enabled me to reflect what I noticed back to the participant more directly, and it enabled participants to reflect on what these multiple co-existing subjectivities meant to them.

Towards the end of the interviews, I checked in with participants to ask how they had experienced the interview process and how they felt at the end. In part, the check-ins were because I adopted an ethic of care and wanted to check how participants felt after the interview to avoid leaving something feeling open or raw. On reflection, the opportunity to reflect also revealed something about the storytelling process for participants. Some participants explained that they were uncertain about how they would feel after sharing their stories, as some had never told them to another person before. Most participants thanked me for the opportunity to talk and for listening to their childhood accounts. Most said that they felt heard or that a weight had been lifted. Some participants explained the emotional and psychological relief they felt at having told their story without being broken down by it and that they felt empowered.

Thinking narratively

I use the term 'thinking narratively' here to situate what follows in this book within narrative inquiry as a research methodology. For the research I conducted, I used a narrative approach to explore young women's narrations of domestic violence. In my view, narrative as a methodology is a tricky, beautiful and diverse terrain to travel. Narrative inquiry is known for being theoretically diverse, fluid and flexible, and there is not a 'one size fits all' approach (Livholts & Tamboukou, 2015). This diversity offers opportunities for researchers to find ways of navigating narrative inquiry in unique and creative ways that are suitable for their own values and the ontologies and epistemologies of their research. I felt that narrative inquiry was particularly useful for this study as it typically aims to centralise voice(s) and engage with issues of relationality and power (Riessman, 2008). There are very limited guides for 'how to do' narrative analysis – mainly because there is no 'one way'. This is one of the beautiful and creative opportunities that narrative analysis can offer researchers: the opportunity to delve into the ontological and epistemological underpinnings of your work and find ways of working with data in a way that feels aligned with values and philosophies that are central to the work.

A point of division within narrative research has been historically characterised by a focus on either (a) experience-led storytelling or (b) socially/culturally and discursively grounded storytelling (Andrews et al., 2013). Feminist narrative scholars have challenged the division of the individual and social from the premise that the stories we tell are both individual *and* socially located (Fraser & MacDougall, 2017; Livholts & Tamboukou, 2015; Mauthner, 2017; Woodiwiss et al., 2017). Consequently, a third relational and dialogical strand of narrative research emerged (Andrews et al., 2013), which places epistemic value on multiple subjectivities and storylines.

A feminist dialogical approach

To understand the participants' stories, I analysed the interview data using a feminist dialogical approach. In this section of the chapter, I outline what a feminist dialogical approach meant in my research and how I worked with the interview data to produce research findings.

It might be useful to summarise how I understand feminism, as I defined previously in Chapter 3. I outlined that feminisms are diverse, plural and locally and socio-culturally located, as well as shaped by each of our individual histories, values and beliefs. Feminist work, thinking and being, as best as I can describe it in the context of my work here, means living feminism as a life question in an effort to work toward a more just and equal world. It means a deep centring and prioritisation of relationships and a recognition that individual lives are embedded in power relations, social systems and legacies of histories. As such, the psychological – that is, our personal experiences and sense of who we are and how we embody ourselves and inhabit spaces – is political. I am particularly interested in the diverse ways we might refuse and rebel against things that have harmed and diminished us. These understandings of feminism guide how I have worked with women's stories in this research.

Drawing on a narrative approach, as described above, I developed a multi-layered approach to listening to young women's stories, which I outline below. To help me do this, I was guided by Arthur Frank's (2012) set of 'commitments' for doing dialogical narrative analysis. Frank's commitments for doing dialogical narrative analysis do not clearly translate to a 'guide' or an analytical strategy, but they have informed my approach to analysis because of his emphasis on voice, multivocality and unfinalisability. These are as follows:

1 To recognise that any individual voice is a dialogue between voices.
2 To remain suspicious of the opposite of dialogue, which is monologue, analysis is not the pursuit of 'truth' or authentic 'voice', but it is the focus on hearing collective voices in dialogue.

3 That stories have 'independent lives' – they are both subjective (belong to the storyteller) and they are external (no story is entirely 'mine' as it is constituted of 'other' voices and forces too; i.e., it is 'borrowed in parts') (p. 36).
4 That humans are 'unfinalised' (p. 36) – that humans have the capacity to grow, change, re-story the self and revise their 'self-understanding', and stories do not necessarily have an 'ending' (pp. 36–37).
5 Refraining from summarising findings or implying the end point of conversation or analysis. Clearly, it is not entirely possible to refrain from summarising findings when writing a book that, at some point, becomes a static offering for others to read. However, I hope that my writing offers a sense of openness to remain curious about continuous sense-making and analytical possibilities and curious about the ways that our own development and growth as listeners will shape how we listen and what we hear; therefore, this book is written with a knowing that there may always be new and different meanings to be heard.

To work with the data, I wanted to find a theoretical frame that would support me in engaging with voice(s) as multiple and stories as polyvocal. I was drawn to Hubert Hermans' Dialogical Self Theory (Hermans, 2001, 2003, 2022). Dialogical Self Theory views selfhood as multiple and dynamic, existing of many voiced 'I positions' that exist in relation to one another. I was drawn to this theory because it seemed to capture something useful in recognising voice as multiple, and it engages with both the unique personal stories of people and the way story and experience are always situated in social, cultural and historical contexts. Bakhtin's (1981) theorisation of space, place and time is central to the dialogical self, proposing that the telling of stories is not a direct expression of the experience itself. Rather, what we talk about and how we tell stories is located and re-constructed across different spaces, places and times.

Hermans' Dialogical Self Theory is informed by Bakhtin's (1981) proposal that the 'I', or subjectivities, have the 'possibility to move from one spatial position to another in accordance with changes in situation and time' (Hermans, 2001, p. 188). Framed in this way, the dialogical model assumes that the self is constituted of many 'selves', which are fluid and dynamic. The 'I' can fluctuate among different, sometimes contradictory positions, and the self is storied through multiple I-positions. Each position is voiced in some way, enabling dialogical relations to be established between these positions. According to Hermans (2001), these voices 'function like interacting characters in a story, involved in a process of question and answer, agreement and disagreement. Each of them has a story to tell about his or her own experiences from his or her own stance' (Hermans, 2001, p. 188).

Dialogical Self Theory considers storytelling as central to how the self is constructed and re-constructed across different times and places. The dialogical approach suggests that the self is narratively constructed through multiple subjective speaking positions. Further, it proposes that it is not just the speaker who shapes how they tell their stories, but importantly, the stories we tell are also shaped by the contexts in which we speak. It is a model of the self that de-individualises the stories we tell by attending to the audience and the context of the speaking, as well as attending to who is doing the speaking (Frank, 2012; Hermans, 2008). Specific to the dialogical approach is the idea that knowledge can be produced at the intersections of voices – by exploring the dialogue *between* voiced subjectivities and *within* the specific contexts in which these subjectivities are voiced (Frank, 2005; Hermans, 2003, 2022). This seemed to align closely with my understanding of feminism, which was to be deeply interested in the personal–political intersections and the way in which individual stories and experiences and social, political and historical contexts are inseparable.

Drawing on Dialogical Self Theory, my analysis of interviews with women in this research was guided by three key assumptions about dialogical selfhood and storytelling. These three key assumptions are listed below.

1. The-other-in-self

'The-other-in-self' refers to the idea that the stories we tell are never entirely our own; rather, some are shaped by cultural and historical contexts, sometimes referred to as narrative resources. Hermans proposes that the operation of power is central to how social, cultural and historical contexts shape how we construct a sense of self. The dialogical model conceptualises the self as constructed by multiple co-existing and voiced I-positions. An 'I' position refers to a speaking position that generally starts with an 'I' statement, such as 'I am…', 'I feel…'. In this book, I also refer to an 'I' position as a 'voice'. These include both 'internal' and 'external' voices (Hermans, 2008). A focus on both internal and external voices enables a focus on how socio-cultural and political contexts shape the stories that we tell about who we are. Framed in this way, it is a model of the self that is not restricted to 'inner voices' only, but that captures 'external voices' too (Hermans, 2001, p. 252).

An emphasis on both internal and external forces enables a focus on how both are interrelated and how individual stories are always situated in and among current and historical power structures. He proposes that this is an identity question, and, instead of the typical question 'Who am I?', a dialogical-informed question would be: 'who am I in relation to the other', and 'Who is the other in relation to me?'. As this is about 'self-in-relation-to-other' rather than a single unitary 'I', there is a recognition that 'I' is always fluid and in-flux, and as such, continuity and discontinuity is key. That is, who we are in relation to our contexts is always open to change, responding to cultural and relational shifts and changes. 'I' is therefore unfinalisable.

2. Multiplicity in unity and de-centralisation of self-knowledge

Multiplicity and the de-centralisation of self-knowledge refer to the idea that the self is multivocal and always in dialogue, rejecting the idea of a single unitary core self. This has also been termed the 'flexibility of "I"' (Hermans, 2022). Hermans highlights how it this theory of the self explicitly rejects the idea that the 'self' is unitary (that is, it is a single, undivided clearly boundaried unit). He explicitly rejects a Cartesian dualistic worldview (that is, that 'self' is separate to and different from society, and that mind and body are two distinctly separate systems) (Hermans, 2003, 2022). As above, this is an identity question that, in his 2022 book, Hermans elaborated that space is an important contextual factor, so the questions become not only 'Who am I in relation to other?' and 'Who is other in relation to me?' but also 'Where am I?'. This space is the physical space I occupy and also the virtual inner space (how I am speaking to myself; what my imagined audience is; what is my inner landscape doing, even when I am alone; who am I imagining is infront of me?), and, how does this space shape the 'I' that comes to the foreground?

The inseparability of 'selves' has been argued consistently by feminist scholars (Choo & Ferree, 2010; Crenshaw, 1991; Staunæs, 2003). Attending to these voices and stories, and also attending to voices that are less likely to be heard, can help to understand how people negotiate the world and the self. Embracing multiplicity means challenging the idea of a single authentic voice – or at least challenging the individualised ontology that the notion of 'authentic voice' is grounded in (Doucet & Mauthner, 2008; Nencel, 2014; Van Stapele, 2014). The research I discuss in this book explores the relationship and dialogue between multiple speaking positions, rather than questioning or interrogating the accuracy of memories themselves.

3. Innovation of self

'Innovation' refers to the idea that humans have the capacity to change, innovate and renew always. This can happen in three ways, according to Hermans (2003). First, it can be when a new position is introduced into the system and leads to a re-organisation of the self (for example, a new role in a family such as mother or daughter, or when playing role play with a child, a new position is introduced and can be flexibly drawn on or 'played' when needed). Second, it can be when there is a re-organisation of already existing positions, for example, if a position moves from background to foreground in a particular situation. For example, a historical or younger part of the self might be backgrounded but in particular instances it might be activated and bought to the foreground. Third, it can be when two or more already existing positions form a cooperation and support each other to form a different or new position; a coalition of positions, of sorts. For example, 'I as playful and free' and 'I as a serious adult' may not have joined forces in a supportive way in the past and may indeed have acted in opposition. However, they may form a coalition through 'I as a poet' or 'I as a photographer'. Innovation as such refers to the idea that 'I' is unstable and always fluid and open to change through re-organisations of 'self'.

Feminist listening

Dialogical Self Theory views dialogue as generative and as a meaning-making project of identity construction and re-construction. Stories are a central part of this. Engaging with storytelling as polyvocal in this way was particularly necessary for this study about experiences of violence. As feminist scholars have noted, when women talk about abuse or violence, their accounts risk being flattened, neglecting the multiplicity of women's stories and identities (Alcoff, 2018; Woodiwiss, 2007), and I consider this the case for accounts of childhood domestic abuse. The dominant focus in existing research tends to be an interest in neatly categorising distress and examining risk and protective factors to determine resiliency or harm because of violence (Levell, 2022). While it is evidently important to take seriously the ways that people can develop resources and strengths and be seriously harmed by violence, it is problematic to assume a logic of binary categorisation when understanding lives that are not experienced or lived in a binary way. As such, this dialogical approach aligned well with a feminist and plural ontology and epistemology that embraces and conceptualises voice as situated (Haraway, 1988), resisting the concept of 'authentic voice' (Nencel, 2014; Van Stapele, 2014), and embracing voice as an 'unstable process' (Chadwick, 2020, p. 6). A dialogical approach to narrative felt useful for this study as it supported a resistance to a binary logic. It felt important that the analysis could attend to not only accounts of strength or struggle, or vulnerability or resilience, in the face of violence, but also to engage with the idea that the self is in motion and unfinalisable; constantly being constructed and re-constructed, both shaped by, and shaping the stories we tell (Gilligan & Eddy, 2021). This commitment to multiplicity meant I could listen for not just one story of childhood domestic abuse, but to listen for many voiced accounts, understanding voice(s) as relational, cultural, embodied and co-constructed.

Working with the Listening Guide and creating and working with voice poems

After transcribing interviews, I used the Listening Guide (Gilligan, 2015) to support analysis. The Listening Guide is a three-phase feminist voice-centred relational method (Brown & Gilligan, 1993; Gilligan & Eddy, 2021). It is a commitment to listening openly, curiously and non-hierarchically. It consists of three 'listenings' whereby the researcher focuses the analysis on a distinct aspect. The listenings are relational, analytical, reflexive engagements with transcripts and audio recordings, so in this sense, 'listening' means more than simply listening to an audio file. The Listening Guide is said to support the researcher to shift from reading the transcript to listening more deeply to the multiple layers of voiced accounts by resisting a binary logic of coding and a hierarchical way of privileging one voice over others (Harel-Shalev & Daphna-Tekoah, 2021).

The first listening is where the researcher listens for the plot. This is where I listened for what was happening in the story, who the key characters were and key moments that the participants highlighted. This was also a reflexive listening where I listened for myself in participants' accounts, and I noted points where I recognised parts of myself or aspects that resonated with me. The second listening is where the researcher listens for the 'I'. This is where I produced I poems. I broke the transcript down into poems; each time a new 'I statement' began in the transcript, I started a new line of a poem, including the 'I', the verb and some of the words that followed that contextualised the 'I' statement. When the 'I' shifted direction, I began a new stanza of the I poem. This resulted in the production of multiple poems from single transcripts where each line marked a new 'I' statement, and each stanza, where the 'I' shifted direction or positionality. I also noticed that sometimes the 'I' was not used, and instead, the second person voice, 'you' was used. In these cases, I included the 'you' in the poems. The final listening is listening for contrapuntal voices; for instance, where multiple voices are expressed that communicate tensions, or contradictory positions. The Listening Guide spoke well to a dialogical philosophy (Hermans, 2001), recognising that the self is not a single unitary subject, but rather, selfhood is dialogical, that is, constituted by an orchestration of multiple voices and selves (Lenz Taguchi, 2012). It directs researchers to attend to the unexpected with curiosity, and it directs researchers to become familiar with people's inner worlds as they are storied through different voices (Gilligan & Eddy, 2021).

The Listening Guide is 'a way to gain access to knowledge or experiences that are dissociated from conscious awareness, and also, on a more theoretical basis, establish the validity of such knowledge' (Gilligan & Eddy, 2021, p. 146). As such, I considered it a valuable epistemic practice, recognising, as discussed in Chapter 3, that epistemic injustices are deeply written into the historical, political and social contexts within which women give voice to experiences of violence. This relational and non-hierarchical way of listening to voices considers 'voice' as psyche that is embedded in body, language and culture. The Listening Guide is based on three assumptions:

- Voice is embodied, meaning voice is expressed through non-verbal communications such as tones, vibrations, sound and breath. It is recognised that voice is part of the physical world we inhabit.
- Voice is in language, meaning that voice is embedded in our social and cultural worlds.

– Voice is a tool of the psyche; that is, voice is about our soul, self and sense of being. This is an understanding that voice is about identity and provides a capacity to communicate something about our experience and who we are.

The three listenings formed the basis for interpretation and analysis. Informed by Frank's (2012) approach to dialogical narrative analysis, I took notes on which narrative resources I saw as shaping each voice, engaging with the contrapuntal voices and the dialogue between voices. I read and re-read the poems and my notes, circling back to questions concerning what narrative resources were shaping what was being said and how, how voices exist in relation with and to each other and what kinds of stories were being voiced through these dialogical orchestrations of voices. I remained interested in how useful these stories were, and to whom.

Developing typologies

Once I had used the Listening Guide and created voice poems, the final stage of analysis was to develop narrative typologies. This was not an effort to develop themes; rather, the purpose was to explore how certain stories shared similar qualities or effects or contained similar storytelling strategies (Frank, 2012). As I outlined in the introductory chapter, the three main research questions guiding this research were: (a) How do women narrate their transitions to young adulthood following domestic violence in childhood? (b) What are the narrative resources that shape how women tell their stories? and (c) How do women construct the self in and through the stories they tell?

I held these questions closely as I developed the typologies. Arthur Frank's (2012) guidance for developing typologies was particularly helpful because he encourages the listener/researcher to be open and curious about how certain stories may be simultaneously useful and limiting for those who tell them. Importantly, a typology does not presume a finite version of the story; it is a recognition that lives are storied and that stories can change. The use of typologies is not intended to be a method of classifying people's stories, as classification can be constraining and finite and restricts opportunities for innovation and possibilities for the self to be storied differently as different positionings become available (Bakhtin, 1981; Frank, 2012). Nor is the use of typologies an assumption that these typologies are 'truth' (Frank, 2012, pp. 14–15). He also proposed that dialogical narrative analysis 'circles back, repeatedly, to asking this question: How well served are people by their stories?' (Frank, 2012, p. 15). I remain close to this question in the three typology chapters that follow.

To develop typologies, I read the transcripts and voice poems multiple times and began writing early in the process. I used pen and paper to construct visual maps that noted key stories and prevalent voices across the dataset. Through deeper reflexive engagement with the women's accounts, I finalised which typologies I felt best represented my understanding of the data. I developed three narrative typologies, 'Transitions', 'Recoveries' and 'Precarious work', which are presented in the following three chapters.

Summary and orientation to the research findings chapters

This chapter has outlined my approach to the research, including how I recruited and interviewed participants and what drew me to use a feminist dialogical approach to analysing the interview data. I have discussed how a dialogical approach was aligned well with feminist ontology and epistemology. I have also explored why I felt it was crucial to engage with voice as multiple and turn an analytical lens to both the individual story and the contexts within which we tell stories about who we are and our life experiences.

In the following three chapters, I discuss the research findings. I use extracts from interview transcripts, and you will find that some of these extracts include my own responses in dialogue with the participant. Including these interactions is necessary to contextualise the data and show how my responses and questions as the interviewer played a role in shaping what the participant said and how.

You might notice that I do not draw on every participant in each chapter. The examples from the interviews I have included reflect the larger dataset as best I can. I use case examples to provide sufficient space to engage with the contextual and relational context of the storytelling in each interview. Therefore, you will find that I sometimes slow down and spend time examining the context of the interview and the relationship between myself and the participant to understand what is being said more. Exploring context in analysis was important. Where I felt it relevant, reflexivity is embedded into the analysis, guided by the assumption that knowledge is relationally and contextually produced. First, I assume that knowledge is produced in local contexts (direct interviewer–interviewee relational spaces), and second, in social/cultural contexts (shaped by broader social and cultural narrative resources) (Hydén, 2013; Mishler, 1986; Phoenix, 2013).

Creating and working with the poems got me curious about staying with the tensions, ambiguities and difficulties of making sense of what appeared contradictory or aspects that, on first listening, did not make sense. I found that important knowledge can be generated by 'staying with' the difficulty (Chadwick, 2021) and by staying with the words in (and in between) the lines of the poems. I include the poems alongside transcript extracts to demonstrate the process of knowledge generation and analysis and to retain the context of the words that wrap around the poems.

The language used in the following chapters is also important to define. I draw on concepts of credibility, coherency and stability. I do not use these words to imply that women themselves lack these qualities. These are terms that I use to talk about the function of the narratives rather than place a particular meaning or judgement on the way that women spoke. It is common that when women talk about trauma or abuse experiences, they risk being misjudged as lacking credibility, stability or reliability. I intend to show that these assumptions are socially and politically located and can powerfully shape how women voice their stories.

References

Alcoff, L. (2018). *Rape and resistance*. Polity Press.
Andrews, M., Squire, C., & Tamboukou, M. (2013). *Doing narrative research* (2nd ed.). SAGE Publications.
Bakhtin, M. (1981). *The dialogic imagination: Four essays*. University of Texas Press.
Braun, V., Clarke, V., & Gray, D. (2017). *Collecting qualitative data: A practical guide to textual, media and virtual techniques*. Cambridge University Press.
Brown, L. M., & Gilligan, C. (1993). Meeting at the crossroads: Women's psychology and girls' development. *Feminism & Psychology*, 3(1), 11–35. https://doi.org/10.1177/0959353593031002
Chadwick, R. (2020). Methodologies of voice: Towards posthuman voice analytics. *Methods in Psychology*, 2. https://doi.org/10.1016/j.metip.2020.100021
Chadwick, R. (2021). On the politics of discomfort. *Feminist Theory*, 22(4), 556–574. https://doi.org/10.1177/1464700120987379
Choo, H. Y., & Ferree, M. M. (2010). Practicing intersectionality in sociological research: A critical analysis of inclusions, interactions, and institutions in the study of inequalities. *Sociological Theory*, 28(2), 129–149. https://doi.org/10.1111/j.1467-9558.2010.01370.x
Crenshaw, K. (1991). Mapping the margins: Intersectionality, identity politics, and violence against women of color. *Stanford Law Review*, 43(6), 1241–1299. https://doi.org/10.2307/1229039
Doucet, A., & Mauthner, N. S. (2008). What can be known and how? Narrated subjects and the Listening Guide. *Qualitative Research*, 8(3), 399–409. https://doi.org/10.1177/1468794106093636
Frank, A. (2005). What is dialogical research, and why should we do it? *Qualitative Health Research*, 15(7), 964–974. https://doi.org/10.1177/1049732305279078
Frank, A. (2012). Practising dialogical narrative analysis. In J. A. Holstein & J. F. Gubrium (Eds.), *Varieties of narrative analysis* (pp. 33–52). SAGE Publications.
Fraser, H., & MacDougall, C. (2017). Doing narrative feminist research: Intersections and challenges. *Qualitative Social Work: Research and Practice*, 16(2), 240–254. https://doi.org/10.1177/1473325016658114
Gilligan, C. (2015). The Listening Guide method of psychological inquiry. *Qualitative Psychology*, 2(1), 69–77. https://doi.org/10.1037/qup0000023
Gilligan, C., & Eddy, J. (2021). The Listening Guide: Replacing judgment with curiosity. *Qualitative Psychology*, 8(2), 141–151. https://doi.org/10.1037/QUP0000213
Grzanka, P. R. (2018). Intersectionality and feminist psychology: Power, knowledge, and process. In C. B. Travis, J. W. White, A. Rutherford, W. S. Williams, S. L. Cook, & K. F. Wyche (Eds.), *APA handbook of the psychology of women* (pp. 585–602). American Psychological Association.

Haraway, D. (1988). Situated knowledges: The science question in feminism and the privilege of partial perspective. *Feminist Studies, 14*(3), 575. https://doi.org/10.2307/3178066

Harel-Shalev, A., & Daphna-Tekoah, S. (2021). Breaking the binaries in research – The Listening Guide. *Qualitative Psychology, 8*(2), 211–223. https://doi.org/10.1037/QUP0000201

Hermans, H. J. M. (2001). The dialogical self: Toward a theory of personal and cultural positioning. *Culture & Psychology, 7*(3), 243–281. https://doi.org/10.1177/1354067X0173001

Hermans, H. J. M. (2003). The construction and reconstruction of a dialogical self. *Journal of Constructivist Psychology, 16*(2), 89–130. https://doi.org/10.1080/10720530390117902

Hermans, H. J. M. (2008). How to perform research on the basis of dialogical self theory? Introduction to the special issue. *Journal of Constructivist Psychology, 21*(3), 185–199. https://doi.org/10.1080/10720530802070684

Hermans, H. J. M. (2022). *Liberation in the face of uncertainty. A new development in dialogical self theory*. Cambridge University Press.

Hollway, W., & Jefferson, T. (2000). *Doing qualitative research differently: Free association, narrative and the interview method*. SAGE Publications.

Hydén, M. (2013). Narrating sensitive topics. In M. Andrews, C. Squire, & M. Tamboukou (Eds.), *Doing narrative research* (2nd ed.) (pp. 223 – 239). SAGE Publications.

Josselson, R. (2013). *Interviewing for qualitative inquiry: A relational approach*. Guilford Press.

Lenz Taguchi, H. (2012). A diffractive and Deleuzian approach to analysing interview data. *Feminist Theory, 13*(3), 265–281. https://doi.org/10.1177/1464700112456001

Levell, J. (2022). *Boys, childhood, domestic abuse and gang involvement*. Bristol University Press.

Livholts, M., & Tamboukou, M. (2015). *Discourse and narrative methods: Theoretical departures, analytical strategies and situated writings*. SAGE Publications.

Mauthner, N. S. (2017). The listening guide feminist method of narrative analysis: Towards a posthumanist performative (re)configuration. In J. Woodiwiss, K. Smith, & K. Lockwood (Eds.), *Feminist narrative research: Opportunities and challenges* (pp. 65–91). Palgrave Macmillan UK.

Mishler, E. G. (1986). *Research interviewing: Context and narrative*. Harvard University Press.

Nencel, L. (2014). Situating reflexivity: Voices, positionalities and representations in feminist ethnographic texts. *Women's Studies International Forum, 43*, 75–83. https://doi.org/10.1016/j.wsif.2013.07.018

Phoenix, A. (2013). Analysing narrative contexts. In M. Andrews, C. Squire, & M. Tamboukou (Eds.), *Doing narrative research*. SAGE Publications.

Riessman, C. K. (2008). *Narrative methods for the human sciences*. SAGE Publications.

Staunæs, D. (2003). Where have all the subjects gone? Bringing together the concepts of intersectionality and subjectification. *NORA - Nordic Journal of Feminist and Gender Research, 11*(2), 101–110. https://doi.org/10.1080/08038740310002950

Tamboukou, M. (2008). Re-imagining the narratable subject. *Qualitative Research, 8*(3), 283–292. https://doi.org/10.1177/1468794106093623

Taylor, S. (2010). *Narratives of identity and place*. Routledge.

Van Stapele, N. (2014). Intersubjectivity, self-reflexivity and agency: Narrating about "self" and "other" in feminist research. *Women's Studies International Forum, 43,* 13–21. https://doi.org/10.1016/j.wsif.2013.06.010

Woodiwiss, J. (2007). Politics, responsibility and adult victims of childhood sexual abuse. *Sociological Research Online, 12*(2), 1–12. https://doi.org/10.5153/sro.1404

Woodiwiss, J., Smith, K., & Lockwood, K. (2017). *Feminist narrative research: Opportunities and challenges*. Palgrave Macmillan UK.

5
TRANSITIONS

I don't know
I don't know if it was a hormonal thing
I don't know
... maybe I just grew up
I just grew up immediately.
I had this very real realisation
I was a grown-up
I needed to cope with stuff
I was still really young
~ Voice poem created from the interview with Clara

Introduction

This chapter is the first of three exploring my research interview analysis. It is about how women spoke about change. Participants' accounts included stories of doing things differently, growing up and how they imagined, hoped or feared their futures.

Dominant narrative resources about developmental transitions – in other words, transitions from childhood to adulthood – assume that child-to-adult development is linear and marked by age (Walkerdine, 1993; Zittoun, 2007). I draw on Tania Zittoun's (2007) socio-cultural relational theory of transitions and change in this chapter. She conceptualises transitions as fluid, unfinalisable and ongoing identity work and development processes shaped by socio-culturally available symbolic resources. As such, when I discuss

DOI: 10.4324/9781003393160-5

narrative 'resources', I refer to these socio-cultural assumptions, ideas and understandings, which shape how participants spoke.

This chapter explores the narrative resources that shaped young women's accounts of transitioning to and navigating young adulthood. I discuss that while age-based and dominant psychological, social and cultural understandings of childhood and adulthood shaped how women narrated their stories, these were both useful *and* limiting. This chapter addresses how women I interviewed spoke about transitions to motherhood and transitions to intimate partner relationships in adulthood and provided accounts of re-negotiating power, authority and voice in young adulthood. It discusses the narrative resources that can simultaneously offer hope as well as limit what can be said and how.

Transitions to motherhood

Some participants spoke about transitions to motherhood. For example, Bethany was studying for her PhD, and had a husband and a child. For all her childhood, she experienced her father's physical and emotional violence towards her mother. When I was interviewing Bethany, one of the key identity transitions that shaped her story was that of becoming a mother:

> I think I've been really focusing on making a home, you know. I've moved around my whole life and the whole of my 20's really. Every year or two just going here or there and I think now, since I've had my daughter I've moved to the place my husband's from... It's a very rural, quiet like, regular life. He had a really regular life and I think that's probably why I picked him. you know, and I'm trying to give them what I, you know, what my idea is of a normal – live in the same house forever, it's really safe and homely and you measure your height on the doorway. You know, that's what I mean.

For Bethany, becoming a mother was told through an account of learning how to 'make a home' with little guidance, and in the aftermath of moving around for her whole life, suggesting a sense of instability. The transition to new motherhood, alongside the model of 'normality' and 'regularity' her husband offered, offered narrative possibilities for change:

> I don't know what to do... when you have a baby people are like oh just do what your mum did, you know, and copy your older relatives. And I think if you don't have a good relationship or a traditional relationship with your older female relatives, you can't because you don't have anything to copy. You know, I find myself reading loads about parenting and I felt really lost. Well, I didn't have the ideal childhood and I don't know

what to copy. I don't know how to do this or how to make a home, and so I found it like a massive learning curve to almost fake it, you know. So I'm in that process, it's becoming real as time goes on - the more I act as if it is. But it's certainly been a process of pretending what you think a regular family is like, you know, just my childhood was not regular. I think I've really been aware since I've had [child] that [parenting] doesn't come naturally.

Feeling overwhelmed when becoming a mother is common (Vincent et al., 2010), and feminist scholars have argued that binary notions of 'good' and 'bad' mothering fail to recognise the reality that most mothers are somewhere in between or that they are both (Oberman & Josselson, 1996). However, becoming a mother had a particular meaning when storied with a history of childhood domestic violence and lack of a mothering guide. Bethany attributed being lost in motherhood to her lack of a 'regular' childhood. The voice poem I made indicates a voice of lostness and a voice of learning:

I don't know what to do
You know
I think
you can't
you don't have anything to copy
you know
I find myself reading loads about parenting
I felt really lost
I didn't have the ideal childhood
I don't know what to copy
I don't know how to do this
I found it like a massive learning curve
I'm in that process, it's becoming real
I act as if it is.

The voice poem shows intersecting voices of lostness ('I felt really lost... I don't know what to copy'), learning ('I find myself reading loads'... 'I found it like a massive learning curve') and hope for change ('I'm in that process, it's becoming real...'). In the narrative surrounding the poem's text, Bethany's story of becoming a mother was shaped by gendered narrative resources that equate femininity with mothering. Her account frames mothering as femininity (Choi et al., 2007; Morell, 2000) by locating 'good' mothering as dependent upon having older women relatives to copy. It is also shaped by the idea that mothering is natural (Ulrich & Weatherall, 2000) through her account of perceived deficit – that mothering does not come naturally to her, and as such, she has to read parenting books and 'pretend' to know what 'regular' family life is like so that her lack of natural expertise is not the reason for her failing. Bethany emphasised the value of competency and knowledge, suggesting that a self-driven success type of narrative resource is useful, as this can enable stories of change and transformation that are read as valuable and position her as having done well. At the same time, this 'success' story may not always make space for articulating ongoing struggle or uncertainty.

The voice poem shows the intersecting narrative resources that shape the dialogical relationship between voices in Bethany's account. One of the key aspects of the dialogical self is the notion of the 'other in self' – the idea that stories have independent lives; they are told both independently *and* they are also told through dialogues we have participated in before. In Bethany's story of becoming a mother, narrative resources of adulthood responsibility and individualising neoliberal values of self-improvement and self-determined 'success' (Gill & Scharff, 2011; McRobbie, 2004, 2015) were powerful in shaping the availability of I positions. For example, by reading parenting books, learning on the job and 'faking it', Bethany's story was shaped by these individualising discourses of self-work and self-improvement.

A transition narrative is limiting in part, but it also does something useful. A further aspect of the dialogical self is recognising the human capacity for innovation. Becoming a mother has introduced a new identity position, a new voice from which to speak and the opportunity for innovation. A new identity as a mother is positioned as Bethany's opportunity to re-construct a 'regular childhood' for herself. What is framed as a deficit of her own childhood is re-storied as having the potential to offer her the opportunity to do things differently. From a new mother identity, Bethany re-constructed the self as more emotionally distanced from her childhood. A re-construction like this can be useful in providing a distance that took her away from the instability and violence of her childhood while simultaneously offering a sense of narrative agency about how her future mothering might be. Oberman and Josselson (1996) proposed that becoming a mother is a series of dialectical tensions – they theorise a matrix of tensions, one of which speaks to these findings: simultaneous loss of self and sense of expansion. This loss of self, or distance from a childhood self, also exists alongside potential expansion and innovation, enabling the possibility that childhood violence does not have to lead to adulthood instability.

Like most participants, stories of chaos and instability also framed Nadine's childhood narration. Nadine was a university student. She had experienced multiple kinds of abuse perpetrated by her father, including direct sexual, physical and emotional abuse towards herself and forced watching of her father's abuse of her mother. Nadine was not in a relationship and did not have children. She described dealing with poor mental health in psychiatric hospitals. She described being on an inpatient psychiatric unit, where interactions with a nurse had 'ingrained' worries of turning out like her father, who had perpetrated violence towards her mother and who had perpetrated organised child sexual exploitation, which included Nadine:

> I really struggled with one nurse who would say like, if I was angry she would just say 'well you're just being like your dad now aren't you?' And I just think that was one of the worst things I could have heard at that point... that would make it a bit more ingrained. You're being like him so therefore you're going to turn out like him. And then once when, because I was asking like 'well, if my childhood wasn't normal? What is normal? I wanted to know – not challenging them but I wanted to know what you would normally do with a baby like when they are this age. But then she would say 'well you could never have children' and I said why? She said 'well because you would treat them like you were treated... I took it on as she's right because I wouldn't know how to treat a child. It doesn't mean – I don't think that I'd, I'd hope that I wouldn't have it in me to do what he did. I don't think I'm that sort of person, but to be told that so directly that you should never have children because you'll end up like him and you'll treat them like he did because that's what you think is right... and that's still in there. I still don't feel like I should have children just in case. Just in case that's the trigger point. Maybe I'm not like that for the rest of my life, but what if having this baby turns me into that person.

Underpinning the nurse's words is an assumption of the inevitability of violence in adulthood following violence in childhood. From one voice, Nadine accepted the nurse's 'expert' narrative that she would not know how to treat a child and should not have children. However, Nadine also rejected that narrative through tentative I statements that suggest, 'I don't think... I'd hope... I don't think I'm that sort of person':

> *I took it on as she's right*
> *I wouldn't know how to treat a child*
> *I don't think that I'd –*
> *I'd hope*
> *I wouldn't have it in me to do what he did.*
> *I don't think I'm that sort of person*
> *I still don't feel like I should have children just in case.*
> *(Maybe) I'm not like that.*

Narrative resources around the intergenerational transmission of violence – that she may start to use violence or become a victim herself (Black et al., 2010) – shaped an internalised questioning voice: what if she does become violent like her father? Alongside this, a resistant voice of hope is tentative. Her I statements often start with 'I think' and 'I hope', suggesting this is a voice of uncertainty. This tentativeness and ambiguity point to the challenge of articulating a voice that diverges from expert narratives with epistemological power. While Nadine was no longer in the hospital, the gendered operation of power between patient and professional still threads through her account. Nadine's questioning ('I said why?') diverges from the politeness and compliance that is demanded from women patients to avoid being read as 'difficult' and having their understandable and legitimate emotions or perspectives read as pathology (Ussher, 2013).

It is also possible that within the relational dynamics of the interview, Nadine was perhaps more able to voice the hesitant voice. In the interview context, I was not a professional in an institution that operated through structures of power that positioned me as 'expert' and Nadine as 'difficult' or 'broken'. Also, while I did not disclose my entire personal history during the interview, Nadine and I had discussed it briefly before the interview, and I had disclosed that I had experienced domestic violence as a child, and this was, in part, why I was interested in learning more. During this part of the interview, I was aware that I have had my own experiences of being a patient within mental health systems, and, as I have experienced myself, these systems can feel oppressive, silencing and punitive. Some of my own understanding and experiences likely informed how I reacted to Nadine's account where I listened with my own felt sense of understanding and did not respond with judgement. This may have facilitated a space where this divergent voice of hesitancy and hope could be articulated.

Blueprints and tentative hope

According to the Dialogical Self Theory, the self has the capacity for innovation and renewal (Hermans, 2001, 2022), meaning that the self is not fixed; the self has the capacity to change, and stories can be one way of reconstructing the self by writing the self into and through a different story. In this chapter so far, I have explored how Bethany and Nadine both drew on the idea that childhoods can act as a blueprint for adulthood and that these can be powerful narrative resources that shape how one stories the self. I want to consider now what this idea of a 'blueprint' means alongside the idea that Dialogical Self Theory offers: that 'self' is fluid and constantly has the capacity for change.

Liv was an undergraduate student when I interviewed her. Liv's biological father was violent towards her mother and her older brother throughout her early childhood. When her biological father left, he cut contact, and her mother began a relationship with a new man who Liv described as her stepfather. He had learning disabilities, and Liv explained that her mother started drinking and became emotionally and physically violent towards her stepdad. At this point, Liv's older brother also became violent towards her mother. Liv's stepfather died a few years prior to the interview, and her mum was left dependent on Liv as a carer. Despite these difficulties, Liv wanted to be interviewed because she wanted to know that her experiences could be used to help other people who had been through similar things. She wanted things to be better in the future for others. She also spoke about wanting things to be better in the future for herself. She spoke about several relationships she had been in with men, which she saw as problematic 'red flag' relationships. Liv referenced her neurodivergence and spoke about dealing with money struggles in the context of her working-class background. Like Bethany, Liv referred to learning how to do things differently in adulthood while highlighting a lack of adult role models:

> it does feel like with my real dad being abusive, I have a lot of problems with men and I do have emotionally abusive relationships, you know like it's really dead cold and then they just cut me off. If I'm in a relationship and they won't listen to my feelings or anything, so I have to build it all up, I don't have anyone to confide in. I was in a long-term relationship with someone and he used to self-harm and he'd threaten suicide and he'd be like "I'm gonna cut myself if you don't come here – I'm gonna like, I'm gonna kill myself" and stuff, you know? I didn't see that as being a massive red flag. I feel like the domestic violence growing up has kind of given me no guide to what a healthy relationship should be like and I accept a lot of stuff I shouldn't accept and then I internalise it and blame myself... I'd just go along with it, it was like a sense of security, but I think sometimes when you grow up in dysfunctional households you do seek out dysfunction as well. But then part of me – I don't wanna be in a dysfunctional relationship because it's too much stress, but I think a lot of people seek them out.
>
> *(Liv)*

Liv's voice of hope for change co-existed with her sense of a lack of blueprint or guide for 'healthy' relationships. A resistant voice of hope that rejects the dominant discourse (that dysfunction in childhood means dysfunction in adulthood) exists in dialogue with voices of hopelessness and self-blame. The voice poem below shows some of what this looked like:

> *I'd just go along with it*
> *I think*
> *you grow up in dysfunctional households*
> *you do seek out dysfunction*
> *I don't wanna be in a dysfunctional relationship*
> *I think a lot of people seek them out.*

In Liv's account, the 'I' slipped away, and she used 'you' when providing an account of dysfunction in childhood. She articulated, 'When you grow up in dysfunctional households, you do seek out dysfunction'. The way that the first-person account slips away and 'you' is used to voice the struggle suggests that narrating both struggle and hope is challenging. Liv's statement, 'I don't wanna be in a dysfunctional relationship because it's too much stress', is a voice of hope that introduces the possibility of an unrestricted future self. Hope can also be viewed as a voice of resistance that offers the possibility of a future that is not solely shaped by the idea that her adulthood will mirror the 'damage' of her past. Additionally, it enables the construct of 'healthy relationships' to be used not only to reflect how harmful her childhood experience of violence was but also as a framework that enabled her to re-story a self that can change.

At the same time, her story was also told through an individualising narrative resource, which was sometimes voiced through a voice of self-blame. For example, Liv's account of her boyfriend's threats to kill himself was told through a voice of self-blame as she attributed her boyfriend's threats to her lack of insight at not seeing the 'red flags'. This individualising self-blame voice functions to attribute blame and free men of their accountability for their violence. For example, the self-responsibilising voice centres the 'I': '*I have* emotionally abusive relationships', rather than '*men* are abusive towards me'. Stories of self-responsibility are also shaped by the expectation that women do emotional labour by attending to their own growth through being insightful and doing emotional work on themselves to better themselves (Alcoff, 2018; Woodiwiss, 2007). The narrative resource directs responsibility to the self for making changes, and blames the self, if change is not always possible or articulatable. Storying the attribution of blame through a self-responsibilising voice also had a useful function. It meant that her experience of violence in childhood has alerted her to what is not good and provides a framework for what she does not want for herself in adulthood. From this view, a narrative framework of normative family life and a self-responsibilising voice can offer useful alternative ways to story the self.

Similarly, Emma spoke about navigating relationships in young adulthood with no role models to base her relationships on. Emma's experience of violence in childhood was that her mother used emotional, psychological and financial abuse towards her father. In the interview, Emma spoke about her experiences navigating intimate relationships in her early adult life without having a guide for how to effectively communicate without arguing and shouting:

> I didn't have much to compare it to, to challenge the idea that you know, it [arguing and shouting] might not be right... it didn't really change until I got married - until I was 21 and you kind of learn on the job so to speak,

don't you – and then you think that this isn't really an effective way to communicate to your other half

(Emma)

There are challenges in talking about transitions to young adulthood when these transitions are uncertain and are shaped by multiple voices. For Emma, 'Learning on the job' about how to do things differently was a story that enabled her to write herself into a position of an independent adult who can change and whose adulthood story does not have to be the same as her childhood one. Framed in this way, stories of learning on the job were useful stories to tell as they construct the self as independent and as successfully transitioning to adulthood and parenthood. However, the possibility of telling alternative stories – stories of failing, fear or doubt – are limited as these would not be socially or culturally valuable stories to tell.

I want to also look at how Jasmine spoke about fears of potentially turning out like her father. Jasmine had just graduated at the time of the interview, and we met via video call on Skype for the interview. She experienced her father's violence against her mother. Her father then left her mother and then became violent towards his new female partner. Jasmine described regular weekend visits to her father's house, where she would be subjected to her father's threats and violence against his partner, and Jasmine would regularly be left to 'fend for herself'. She explained that each time she visited, it would have a knock-on impact on the rest of her week once she returned home to her mother, and she would become aggressive and highly anxious at home and school. She attributed this anger to the fear she felt of her father, and she also used these memories as a 'tool' to ensure she would 'not become like that':

> But the anger – [pause] I think the anger I dealt with was I saw him as something that I definitely didn't wanna be. I didn't want to be violent like he was, so I kind of used that as a picture of something that I never wanted to become. So I used my memories as a tool to not become like that… When I used to get angry I used to say to my mum all the time that I'd get scared cos when I was angry I felt like I wanted to hit people all the time. Cos I couldn't - when I was angry, I couldn't show it and I – I had urges to just lash out. So that was something that I really struggled with
>
> *(Jasmine)*

Considered in this way, this story of lacking a role model was storied for Jasmine in a way that became a 'tool' for good. A tool for not being like her father. While this was a struggle, it also seemed to shape a story for Jasmine that centred something positive and a story in which her lack of a positive blueprint or role model in childhood did not necessarily have to imply a lifetime of anger and violence herself.

Getting older and expressions of voice

This section is about how participants narrated transitions through stories that centralised 'getting older' with a greater capacity to 'speak out'. Age is one way that psychology has typically conceptualised developmental transitions (Crafter et al., 2019; O'Dell et al., 2018), with childhood being positioned as a time of 'becoming' an independent and autonomous person. Participants drew on this child–adult binary and linear developmental trajectory when they spoke about growing up, particularly when storying how getting older was associated with speaking up or being taken more seriously.

Sochi was a student at the time of the interview. We met at her university for an in-person interview. She explained that her biological father had separated from her mother when she was very young and that her mother had multiple subsequent male partners who were all violent towards her mother. Sochi lived with her mother and other family members and often experienced financial insecurity. Her mother's partners did not usually live with them, but they would still perpetrate physical and psychological abuse. Sochi recalled an instance when her mother's partner was physically violent as she had turned 16.

> it was my 16th birthday and I was out and I received a call from my mum and she was like 'oh where are you?' and she told me what happened – she had been on the sofa and they were arguing and he dragged her off the sofa, which she then tried to run out of the house, he dragged her back inside the house and got on top of her and was going to punch her but then something clicked and he didn't and then he stormed off out of the house so then she called me. She was like oh he's out, this has happened, etc, I just don't want you to run into him on your way back. So obviously I'd come back and they stayed together after that again. So again it was the whole swallow what I think. And I did say this time, oh what I thought. But again this time, not my place, if that's what you wanna do like, what can I do? But erm, the second time again they'd had an argument, we'd just had dinner. I think I took my plate back to the kitchen and was washing up and then when I came back my mum was like 'oh I can't believe you just did that' and he had whacked her around the head with a newspaper – erm, and I just lost my shit (slight laugh) cos I was just like, oh I'd had enough. Ended up squaring up at him with him right directly in my face. He was swearing at me, and then he just refused to leave. He just went up to the bedroom and refused to leave. So I had to call the police and the police had to come and actually remove him from the property. Erm, so (pause) it got to the point where I did eventually say something and it got to the

point where (pause) obviously being older, erm (pause) it's yeah (pause) easier... it was just at a point where it was like you can't get away with doing this shit. Like, you just can't.

(Sochi)

Through Sochi's account, growing up and getting older enabled space to act by calling the police and 'squaring up' to her mother's partner when she had 'had enough'. One aspect of Sochi's identity as an adult was that she prides herself on being able to speak out and speak up against injustices. She explained this had strengthened as she grew older. Using her voice to speak out was a key feature of her adult identity. In contrast, her childhood was narrated as a time of lacking opportunities to speak out against the abuse or to be taken seriously if she did:

> I just despised the man so much, I just really really did. I think even at that age, I think I just kind of kept my mouth shut and just kind of like got on with it really... I was at an age where I was too young to really be able to speak my opinion on that situation properly... as an adult I find that very very difficult, like I can't ignore things, erm, having done that as a child for so long over so many different things, erm, I now find it almost impossible to ignore things, erm, and just pretend that everything is fine cos obviously I didn't have any say in that.

(Sochi)

As seen above, for Sochi, childhood meant a time when she was 'too young' to speak her opinion 'properly', whereas adulthood, she proceeded to account for, is a time when she cannot 'ignore things'. The voice poem, constructed from the above interview extract, demonstrates this shifting polyvocality from both 'I' positions; 'I as adult' and 'I as child':

> *I think even at that age*
> *I think*
> *I just kind of kept my mouth shut*
> *I was at an age*
> *I was too young to really be able to speak my opinion*
> *I find that very very difficult*
> *I can't ignore things*
> *I now find it almost impossible to ignore things*
> *I didn't have any say in that*

Through her account of adulthood, speaking out and using her voice against injustices is storied as 'almost impossible' not to do. 'I as adult' – the self that speaks out and 'can't ignore things', is narrated in contrast with 'I as child' – who kept her 'mouth shut'. Looking at it in this way, the constraints of childhood are narrated as a struggle, and adulthood is narrated through a liberated 'I'. Drawing on Dialogical Self Theory, the operation of social power can help to understand what is happening here in the dialogical relationship between 'I as adult' and 'I as child'. In Sochi's account, turning 16 appears to have particular social and cultural meanings, including the idea that turning 16 increases the capacity and ability to act, making space for and enabling stories of action and agency. This can be understood as being shaped by social and cultural notions. Childhood is a passive time of 'becoming' rather than children being active agents in their lives (Horton & Kraftl, 2006; Qvortrup, 2009). These notions of childhood shape the discursive ground from which Sochi spoke about growing up and speaking out. Framed in this way, Sochi told a story of speaking out and taking action with the premise that it was her 16th birthday, symbolising getting older and becoming an adult and, consequently, increasing her capacity to take action.

Her story positions the transition to adulthood as pivotal in her capacity to use her voice and take action. Sochi's accounts of staying quiet and speaking out point to a negotiation of power that is temporal and shifts depending on time and age. Narrative resources of adulthood independence enabled Sochi to write herself into a position as a capable, independent adult through the telling of her story, bolstered by the way that childhood is constructed as a time of passivity. For example, being 'too young to speak my opinion properly' speaks to notions of childhood as somehow lacking in rationality and competency. Sochi's account told a story of childhood where she lacked the authority to have a valued opinion and have it taken seriously by adults. As an adult speaker, these stories of growing up offered opportunities for voice and epistemic authority, particularly as adulthood is storied as a time when it is impossible not to stay silent.

Storying the self into a position of autonomy and action through becoming an adult can be useful. Still, a narrative framework of the child-to-adult developmental trajectory and assumed adulthood autonomy and rationality can also be limiting and may not make space for uncertainty, change or other ways of agency and action in childhood. The voice poem I constructed from the interview with Sochi suggests that agency and action in adulthood can be articulated through a voice of being pushed over the edge. In the below voice poem, I have also included where storying 'he' (her mother's partner') intersects with the 'I' to provide context for how 'I' was relating with others:

he had whacked her around the head with a newspaper
I just lost my shit
I'd had enough. Ended up squaring up at him with him right directly in my face.
He was swearing at me

he just refused to leave
He just went up to the bedroom and refused to leave
I had to call the police

The voice of being pushed over the edge is expressed through statements such as: 'I just lost my shit' and 'I'd had enough'. On the surface, this could be understood as a voice of anger. Still, on closer reading, and in the context of a liberated adult 'I', the sense of having lost her 'shit' speaks to a sense of built-up emotions, so much so that they overspill; they leak out, and one loses one's composure. As such, this voice of leaking out and overspilling emotions suggests that it is not only age that was a factor in Sochi's negotiation of power but also the growing emotions she felt about her mother's violent partners over time. Dominant age-based narrative resources of growing up provide a framework through which to tell stories of growing up in a linear way. Still, they do not make space for stories that include other experiences shaped by emotion or relationships. Opportunities to construct the self as agentic before turning 16 are limited due to the age-based narrative framework of child-to-adult development, as there are limited ways to describe these agentic actions in ways that will be heard as legitimate by others. As such, this narrative resource is limited as it constrains the speakability of agency and action in childhood, leading to the potential for these stories of childhood to construct the self as helpless or to blame (McKenzie-Mohr & Lafrance, 2011).

'I' as adult and re-negotiations of power

Re-negotiations of power through storytelling enabled Sochi to tell a story of action and agency, reasserting herself as active and independent in adulthood. The social and cultural power of narrative resources that associate adulthood with independence and maturity were useful in shaping her story, enabling her to write herself into a position of action and of having a voice. In the absence of stories of linear recovery from her experiences, and in the context of a childhood that Sochi emphasised as 'not normal', her position as a young adult who has a voice and speaks out was a central part of her identity, enabling her to reject stories of passivity, self-blame and helplessness.

Other participants also drew on the growing-up narrative resource to talk about their transitions to young adulthood. Clara explained that her ways of coping with the domestic violence changed as she grew older. Clara's father used abuse against her mother, and Clara emphasised the emotional and financial abuse and the ways this continued to haunt her life.

Clara: *I had school which was, you know, trying to cope with all that sort of stuff all of the time, which is still quite stressful for a kid,*

>   on top of all of that. And then I also had [brother], which was
>   kind of like an extra branch to that. There was a lot going on.
>   I guess yeah it was easier to run away than fight it most of the
>   time. Yeah, and it's interesting cos at high school that stopped. All
>   of a sudden I became a teenager and it was like you know, very
>   much reality – I definitely didn't use the escapism route in high
>   school – definitely not.
> Int: do you know what changed for you?
> Clara: ermm I don't know. I don't know if it was a hormonal thing, or…
>   I don't know. Maybe I just grew up. It sort of stopped at like, I
>   was about [pause] I don't know how old you are when you go
>   into year 8? 12 ish. Yeah that's when it all kind of stopped. It was
>   like I just grew up immediately.
> Int: so what stopped?
> Clara: just that escapism. That ability to run away from stuff just stopped.
>   I had this very real realisation that I was a grown-up, and I needed
>   to cope with stuff even though I was still really young.

In Clara's account, growing up was almost 'immediate' and happened 'all of a sudden', *and* at the same time, the lines between child and adult positions blur. Growing up was both immediate and uncertain. I created a voice poem from the above extract to show the interplay between I positions; 'I as grown-up' and 'I as young':

> *I don't know*
> *I don't know if it was a hormonal thing*
> *I don't know*
> *… maybe I just grew up*
> *I just grew up immediately.*
> *I had this very real realisation*
> *I was a grown-up*
> *I needed to cope with stuff*
> *I was still really young.*

The voice poem shows the polyvocality of Clara's account, demonstrating that the self is constructed through multiple co-existing voices that are often contradictory. On the one hand, Clara stated, 'I was a grown-up' and 'I needed to cope with stuff'. From another voice, she also said, 'I was still really young'. Viewed in this way, growing up means you need to 'cope with stuff'; however, there is a challenge in 'growing up' when you are still young ('I was still really young') and things are still difficult ('there was a lot going on'). Dialogical Self Theory (Hermans, 2001, 2022) considers these co-existing voices as 'multiplicity in unity', assuming that the self is not a singular stable 'I' but rather, 'self' is multiple, voiced almost through an orchestration of co-existing, sometimes contradictory, I positions. For Clara, 'I as grown-up' and 'I as still young' exist in dialogue, alongside a hesitant 'I don't know'. The hesitant 'I don't know' indicates a grappling with how to narrate a coherent stable 'I' when 'I' is constituted of voices that do not always align in a way that is heard and read as coherent by others.

Like Sochi, Clara's account was shaped by dominant narrative frameworks about growing up. Adulthood is a narrative resource that offers something useful. It enabled Clara to write herself into a story of coping in 'adult' ways (not using escapism, which is framed as a childlike thing to do). Clara stated, 'I was a grown-up, and I needed to cope with stuff'. However, adulthood only offers limited stories to tell. It can be a constraining narrative resource, particularly when her experience may not align with normative frameworks about what adults are expected to do (i.e. to 'cope with stuff').

Age was a key part of these growing-up stories, and this is not surprising given the social and cultural dominance of age-based developmental stages and the subsequent framing of childhood and adulthood as separate entities (O'Dell et al., 2018). In my analysis of transition stories, growing up was storied as sometimes dependent on age, but not always, and not only. I explored earlier in this section that for Sochi, turning 16 symbolised a greater capacity to act and as such, legitimised 'I as adult'. Similarly, in Clara's account, turning 18 meant she finally had 'no tie' to her father and could be 'done' with him. Clara continued to have contact by visiting her father when she was younger, and she explained how this was traumatic and heightened anxieties, including nightmares, fear and struggles with being at school. She explained the relief she felt when she reached 18 and could decide for herself to cut ties. However, turning 18 did not necessarily mean no more contact. She explained how her father continued to use family courts, withholding money in the face of requests to support her mother financially for caring for her sibling, to maintain contact and maintain control over her, her mother and her sibling:

> Naturally, you go and see your dad. You know, you have contact, it seems the right thing to do in those... I don't wanna say in those days cos it sounds like a really long time ago, and it wasn't. But it did seem like the right thing to do, to go see him, and actually it wasn't. And I think she (mum) felt a lot of pressure from him for us to go see him, so it just became a natural thing for us to go and see him, erm, but it was definitely a release to kind of finally say "I'm done. I don't wanna do this anymore". And even more so at 18 when I finally had no tie to him whatsoever, although I did – cos we asked him for that money. And even now, he's bringing me into it, and I'm not even a part of it
>
> *(Clara)*

Growing up and becoming an adult was marked by turning 18 when Clara decided she did not want to have contact with her father. Her statement of independence exists despite her account that you 'naturally' see your father, and contact seems like the 'right thing to do'. Voices of adulthood autonomy and independence can be seen as a resistance to the taken-for-grantedness and naturalisation of family relationships that have been harmful to her. However, through Clara's account, it was also clear that it was not as simple as deciding not to 'do this anymore'. Clara's ongoing contact with her dad had not stopped just because she turned 18. Her family still needed financial input from him, mainly to contribute to the care of Clara's sibling, who was disabled. Each time her mother asked her father for money, her father refused, Clara suspected, purely to take them to court. As such, Clara explained she then becomes intimately caught up in the dynamics that she wanted to be released from when she decided at 18 that she 'was done'. From this view, growing up is not simply marked by age, but it is relational and complicated to navigate. The voice poem I constructed from Clara's account helps to show the dialogical relationship between voices:

I'm done
I don't wanna do this anymore.
I finally had no tie to him whatsoever
... I did – cos we asked him for that money
he's bringing me into it
I'm not even a part of it

In the poem above, I want to draw attention to the contradictions and inconsistencies between I positions, assuming that these inconsistencies point to sites of knowledge and meaning. From one voice, Clara stated, 'I'm done... I don't wanna do this anymore', 'I finally had no tie to him' and 'I'm not even a part of it'. Through another voice, she articulated, 'I did', and 'he's bringing me into it'. 'I' that has a tie to her father and 'I' that wants nothing to do with her father meet each other in this orchestration of voices. This has a particular meaning in the context of the coercive control she described her father using through the family courts. The story she told was a story of asserting autonomy and independence but through a web of coercive control that her dad still maintained in the family system. The relational context here makes narrating stories of adulthood autonomy and independence challenging; voices of autonomy and independence were compromised by her dad's ongoing abuse and Clara's position in the family as her sibling's carer. Clara occupied multiple I positions, meaning her stories were neither one-dimensional nor consistent. The interplay of voices demonstrates how her account of her transition to young adulthood is dialogically produced.

My analysis of these accounts suggests that the separateness of childhood and adulthood is not easily, and not only, defined by age markers. In the context of coercive control, complex family relationships and domestic violence, transitions to young adulthood are made more complicated to narrate as these contextual and relational circumstances provide constraints and non-normative ways of experiencing family life. However, a binary logic of childhood and adulthood as separate entities still provides a narrative resource through which young women told their stories in ways that were both useful and limiting. For Clara, she 'just grew up' when she was 'still young'. Age-based markers dictated her storytelling, such as becoming a teenager or turning 18. However, her experience of these ages told different stories that do not conform to the narrative framework of what might be expected at these age-based points. For example, she was brought into the family system even though she was an adult and coped in 'grown-up' ways, even when she was still young.

Summary

In this chapter, I have drawn on Dialogical Self Theory (Hermans, 2001, 2022) and Tania Zittoun's socio-cultural relational theory of transitions and change (2007). I have considered transitions as fluid, unfinalisable and ongoing identity work and development processes shaped by socio-culturally available symbolic resources. In providing extracts from interviews and examples of voice poems I created from interview transcripts, I have shown that young women I interviewed storied change and transition in their lives through and after domestic violence as dialogical, negotiated and uncertain processes in which the 'I' is not always stable. New identity positions such as 'I as mother', 'I as adult' or 'I as partner' can provide new and different narrative resources that can support women to narrate themselves through and into new identities that offer hope and possibilities for change. These identity positions can mean that perceived childhood deficits could be re-storied as having the potential to provide opportunities for change. I have also explored how these new identity positions can, at the same time, provide narrative resources that can be constraining and limit the possibilities of what can be voiced.

Gendered and age-based discourses intersect and shape women's accounts. Narrative resources of adulthood, femininity and 'success' enabled women to construct an autonomous self that can change, producing a stable self and an account of the culturally valuable self. However, these narrative resources can also be limiting. In Liv's account, I highlighted a voice of responsibility where she spoke about intimate relationships in adulthood, assuming that she was to blame for not seeing the 'red flags' in her partner. I have explored that self-responsibility in storytelling can offer a sense of agency. Still, these stories are shaped by neoliberal and patriarchal values, in which women who succeed are responsible for their success, and those who don't become accountable for their failures, too (McRobbie, 2004).

This chapter has considered that women can be left with few alternative ways of telling their stories if their experiences do not align with these success stories. The pervasiveness of deficit and damage discourses, especially in the absence of a 'good' blueprint and in the absence of older women role models in the family, become heavily implicated in what stories are available to tell and how. For example, women's mothering capabilities or their 'success' in adulthood were storied as dependent on their childhood blueprints. These stories, shaped by deficit and what was lacking, also consisted of uncertainties, disruption, struggle and shame. 'Success' stories may not make space for these tensions, contradictions and feelings that do not align with how these stories of success 'should' look. Consequently, young women may be simultaneously bolstered and restricted by the neoliberal and patriarchal ideologies that shape their stories of change and transition when navigating early adulthood.

To summarise, developmental transitions, as I understand women's accounts, are not just about what has been in the past but also about how one stories what is yet to come. Developmental transitions for the women I interviewed were not 'complete', suggesting that 'I as adult' is a process rather than a fixed endpoint. There were limited possibilities for women to authorise their biographies, including their stories of the future. Re-storying the self is tentative and uncertain, mainly when the new story includes resistance to expert stories that have been told before about them or about people like them, such as the nurse who told Nadine not to have children 'in case' she turned out like her father. However, stories of transitions can be powerful depending on who is willing to hear and on what kind of narrative resources are available to draw on. Depending on the context of the telling, the self can be written into resistance and hope.

References

Alcoff, L. (2018). *Rape and resistance*. Polity Press.

Black, D. S., Sussman, S., & Unger, J. B. (2010). A further look at the intergenerational transmission of violence: Witnessing interparental violence in emerging adulthood. *Journal of Interpersonal Violence*, 25(6), 1022–1042. https://doi.org/10.1177/0886260509340539

Choi, P., Henshaw, C., Baker, S., & Tree, J. (2007). Supermum, superwife, supereverything: Performing femininity in the transition to motherhood. *Journal of Reproductive and Infant Psychology*, 23(2), 167–180. https://doi.org/10.1080/02646830500129487

Crafter, S., Maunder, R., & Soulsby, L. (2019). *Developmental transitions: Exploring stability and change through the lifespan*. Routledge.

Gill, R., & Scharff, C. (2011). *New femininities: Postfeminism, neoliberalism, and subjectivity*. Palgrave Macmillan.

Hermans, H. J. M. (2001). The dialogical self: Toward a theory of personal and cultural positioning. *Culture & Psychology*, 7(3), 243–281. https://doi.org/10.1177/1354067X0173001

Hermans, H. J. M. (2022). *Liberation in the face of uncertainty. A new development in dialogical self theory*. Cambridge University Press.

Horton, J., & Kraftl, P. (2006). Not just growing up, but going on: Materials, spacings, bodies, situations. *Children's Geographies, 4*(3), 259–276. https://doi.org/10.1080/14733280601005518

McKenzie-Mohr, S., & Lafrance, M. N. (2011). Telling stories without the words: 'Tightrope talk' in women's accounts of coming to live well after rape or depression. *Feminism & Psychology, 21*(1), 49–73. https://doi.org/10.1177/0959353510371367

McRobbie, A. (2004). Post-feminism and popular culture. *Feminist Media Studies, 4*(3), 255–264. https://doi.org/10.1080/1468077042000309937

McRobbie, A. (2015). Notes on the perfect: Competitive femininity in neoliberal times. *Australian Feminist Studies, 30*(83), 3–20. https://doi.org/10.1080/08164649.2015.1011485

Morell, C. (2000). Saying no: Women's experiences with reproductive refusal. *Feminism & Psychology, 10*(3), 313–322. https://doi.org/10.1177/0959353500010003002

O'Dell, L., Brownlow, C., & Bertilsdotter Rosqvist, H. (2018). *Different childhoods: Non/normative development and transgressive trajectories*. Routledge.

Oberman, Y., & Josselson, R. (1996). Matrix of tensions: A model of mothering. *Psychology of Women Quarterly, 20*(3), 341–359. https://doi.org/10.1111/J.1471-6402.1996.TB00304.X

Qvortrup, J. (2009). Childhood as a structural form. In J. Qvortrup, W. A. Corsaro, & M.- S. Honig (Eds.), *The palgrave handbook of childhood studies* (pp. 21–33). Palgrave Macmillan.

Ulrich, M., & Weatherall, A. (2000). Motherhood and infertility: Viewing motherhood through the lens of infertility. *Feminism & Psychology, 10*(3), 323–336. https://doi.org/10.1177/0959353500010003003

Ussher, J. M. (2013). Diagnosing difficult women and pathologising femininity: Gender bias in psychiatric nosology. *Feminism & Psychology, 23*(1), 63–69. https://doi.org/10.1177/0959353512467968

Vincent, C., Ball, S. J., & Braun, A. (2010). Between the estate and the state: Struggling to be a 'good' mother. *British Journal of Sociology of Education, 31*(2), 123–138. https://doi.org/10.1080/01425690903538976

Walkerdine, V. (1993). Beyond developmentalism? *Theory & Psychology, 3*(4), 451–469. https://doi.org/10.1177/0959354393034004

Woodiwiss, J. (2007). Politics, responsibility and adult victims of childhood sexual abuse. *Sociological Research Online, 12*(2), 1–12. https://doi.org/10.5153/sro.1404

Zittoun, T. (2007). Symbolic resources and responsibility in transitions. *YOUNG, 15*(2), 193–211. https://doi.org/10.1177/110330880701500205

6
RECOVERIES

I picture myself as a little girl... that's who I'm talking about
I know
I am that little girl
that isn't me
Although it is
I've lived like two lives
       ~ *Voice poem created from the interview with Jasmine*

Introduction

This is the second chapter that discusses research findings. This chapter focuses on how young women I interviewed narrated their recoveries after childhood domestic violence. I explore the narrative resources women drew on to talk about recovery after domestic violence. These include psychotherapeutic narrative resources that shaped 'successful' recovery stories. It also examines how self-development work and a quest for authenticity were storied as central to some of these 'successful' recovery narratives. I also explore how 'forgiving and forgetting' shaped some participants' accounts and how 'using your story for good' could be a way of narrating a recovery that is socially and culturally valuable. This chapter considers the role of gender and the particular ways that epistemic authority is navigated in the context of childhood domestic violence that was largely unseen and unheard.

DOI: 10.4324/9781003393160-6

Storying the self as a psychotherapeutic subject

In narrating recoveries, I found that some participants' accounts were centred around a pivotal moment of realisation. For example, realisations that they were struggling, realising their childhood was not 'normal' and piecing together parts of their life and making sense of it in ways that they had not done before. I understand these kinds of accounts as shaped by a psychotherapeutic narrative resource and, through this, storying the self as a psychotherapeutic subject. This refers to the way that a story shaped by psychotherapy, psychology or a psychiatric narrative resource offers a way of making sense of and storying the self in a way that may be read as legitimate by others. This kind of psychotherapeutic narrative resource could be both useful and limiting when women spoke about their childhood experiences of domestic violence and recoveries.

Psychotherapeutic narrative resources shaped stories that were characterised by efforts to change, diagnose or understand the self for difficulties to be eased or to live what some participants referred to as 'a better life' or to live more 'authentically'. This kind of self-reflective gaze was one way in which women narrated recovery stories and made meaning out of childhood domestic violence. It was also an important way of enabling women to story a self that has moved on and recovered. For example, Hayley had experienced various traumas in childhood and adolescence, including but not only parental domestic abuse. She had also experienced her own mental health struggles relating to trauma and an eating disorder, and she highlighted her sense that it was likely that she would have gone down the 'path' of mental illness, as she was more 'at risk':

> I had more risk factors that I was going to choose to go down the path that I went, therefore there was more chaos during my adolescence and there was more risk of mental illness
>
> *(Hayley)*

Some of Hayley's interview included her reflections on why she struggled with her mental health, suggesting efforts to explain and make sense of the struggles she had experienced. In doing so, she explained that she grew up on a poor council estate, had young parents and was around drugs and alcohol from a young age, in addition to parental domestic abuse. Through her account, she turned the gaze inwards in a self-reflective way by using statements such as 'I had more risk factors... I was going to choose to go down the path that I went'. I understand this as a self-evaluative structure to her storytelling, drawing on expert language such as 'risk factors'. This self-evaluative structure points to psychotherapeutic and psychiatric discourses that, due to an individualising model of mental illness and health, promote a self-reflective and internalised gaze (Rose, 2010).

Liv, like Hayley, had experienced mental health struggles. In my interview with Liv, she also made efforts to explain and make sense of why she had struggled and continued to struggle so much. Liv had experienced significant physical violence from her biological father and her older brother. When her biological father left the home, her older brother continued to use violence, and her mother then became the perpetrator of violence towards her subsequent partner. During the interview, Liv spoke about experiencing eating disorders, body image difficulties and trauma, and her suspicion that she is also neurodivergent. Her narration was also shaped by similar self-evaluative structures as she spoke about the 'black mark' that she felt she carried due to her childhood experiences:

> I feel like my whole childhood is like a black mark and people can see it – makes me feel dirty and like, different... I really struggle with relationships and friendships and stuff. I'm actually going through an assessment for Asperger's because I feel like, I don't know [pause] I feel like I do score highly on all the tests and stuff and I don't know if it's that, or if it's all the trauma that makes me this way.
>
> *(Liv)*

Liv's uncertainty, 'I don't know if it's that, or if it's all the trauma', points to the challenge she faced in narrating a self that is read and heard as coherent and stable. Efforts to understand herself by making links between childhood trauma and adulthood difficulties threaded through Liv's interview as she made sense of her current struggles by linking them to her past trauma. Liv's inward gaze shows her efforts at making sense of her childhood, but making sense of her childhood is not straightforward. A diagnostic and psychotherapeutic narrative resource enabled possible alternative constructions of the self that were not led by self-blame and shame, and that enabled a legitimised way of making sense of her struggles. Telling her recovery story through this kind of self-evaluative structure made possible a story in which at least her struggles can be recognised, and her own sense of shame might be lightened. However, the voice that is shaped by a sense of carrying a 'black mark' appears to be articulated through 'I as different' and 'I as dirty'. This voice speaks to shame and has a way of constructing the self as permanently 'damaged' due to her childhood experiences. As I discussed in Chapter 2, this voice can be understood as shaped by an academic and social narrative resource of the trajectory of inevitable damage that people who grow up with domestic violence are assumed to experience.

These individualising psychotherapeutic narrative resources also shaped the way that Emma storied recovery, as she also made efforts to make sense of her difficulties. I introduced Emma in Chapter 5, where I explored her account of transitioning to young adult intimate partner relationships, feeling both marked by her lack of a role model in childhood and having to 'learn on the job' about how to be in adult relationships that are not marked by arguing and fighting. During my interview with Emma, she also reflected on the fact that she had self-referred for an Attention Deficit Hyperactivity Disorder (ADHD) assessment, and she considered the similarities and overlap between ADHD and the impacts of trauma. In some ways, she used the interview dialogue as a space to give voice to both self-evaluative and self-pathologising voices alongside a voice of self-compassion and understanding. All these voices exist in dialogue, and point to attempts to understand the self and attribute a reason for her difficulties:

Emma: *I kind of referred myself for an ADHD diagnosis and cos as time's gone on I've kind of learnt about myself and about ADHD and I kind of (pause) don't (pause) really see it in that way (pause).*

Int: *in what way?*

Emma: *I don't want to say (pause) – like I can kind of rationalise my struggles (pause) as something you know – (pause) I just find it interesting that I had to pathologise myself (slight laughter) to give myself an OK, and a reason why I do these things, a reason that I get anxious and a reason that I behave in this way. It's because I've got ADHD. But actually I think now I realise (pause) well I'm trying to remind myself (pause) that maybe I've just had some hard experiences that have made me – that have moulded me in that way.*

The voice poem I constructed from the above interview extract demonstrates some of the polyvocality in Emma's account as she grapples with a self-pathologising voice, a quest to know and understand her struggles and a voice of self-compassion:

I've kind of learnt about myself and about ADHD
I kind of don't really see it in that way
I don't want to say
I can kind of rationalise my struggles
I just find it interesting
I had to pathologise myself to give myself an OK, and a reason why
I do these things
I get anxious
I behave in this way

> *I've got ADHD*
> *I think*
> *I realise*
> *I'm trying to remind myself*
> *(maybe) I've just had some hard experiences that have made me – that have moulded me*

In Emma's efforts to narrate an account of self-understanding, there is a voice of self-compassion: 'I'm trying to remind myself that maybe I've just had some hard experiences'. There is also a voice that she names herself as pathologising: 'It's because I've got ADHD'. At the same time, there is also a voice that rejects this kind of 'pathologising' through self-evaluation: 'as time's gone on I've kind of learnt about myself and about ADHD and I kind of don't really see it in that way'. From this view, while Emma rejected a psychotherapeutic discourse, a diagnosis of ADHD also offers a legitimised way she can story her difficulties. This kind of 'expert' story functioned to authorise Emma's struggles, making her story credible and readable to others. In some ways, this psychotherapeutic narrative resource bolsters the voice of self-compassion by providing a way of understanding herself. At the same time, this way of understanding herself is rejected. There is also an 'I' that does not really see it in 'that way'. As Woodiwiss (2014) has also explored with women who had experienced childhood sexual abuse, this 'pathologisation' can be a route to understanding oneself. However, Emma's rejection of the fact that she had to pathologise herself points to the tension in narrating the reasons for her struggles and the challenge of telling a story that renders her recovery credible.

Emma's negotiation of these tensions continued, as she explained:

> I think I'm learning to be a bit kinder to myself and think, you know I didn't experience you know a rape you know, or an event, but I saw lots of little things over a long period of times… I have to remind myself that that can be quite traumatising.
>
> *(Emma)*

Telling a story through a self-evaluative structure enabled Emma to link the past to the present in a way that made sense, stabilising her story and her 'self' through expert discourses. As I understand Emma's account, it might also be that these psychotherapeutic self-evaluative narrative resources may also enable the possibility for the self to be constructed as someone deserving of kindness and empathy. From one voice, Emma said: 'I'm learning to be kinder to myself' and 'I've held onto it for so long and it tears you apart'. Emma's recovery story told through this psychotherapeutic inward gaze had a way of enabling Emma to re-construct herself as someone who was not responsible for her struggles; she owns them, but through this self-evaluative recovery story, she is not to blame for them.

Examining the socio-cultural contexts in which these stories were told in is important in making sense of them. These stories of efforts to develop self-understanding, with the quest for self-improvement, were told in a neoliberal context that privileges self-driven success and happiness. As such, these are culturally valuable stories to tell, particularly if they help a person to write themselves into a 'survivor' identity (Alcoff & Gray, 1993; Rose, 1985). Neoliberal ideologies can be understood as promoting a self-evaluative structure in which the self is constructed as a therapeutic subject, and the work of recovery is to work on the self in ways that are seen as successful (Woodiwiss, 2014). Storying the self into a position of 'success', or even in the process of the quest for self-understanding and self-development, enables a coherent narrative and offers ways of making sense of distress while also offering solutions to address such distress (i.e. therapy, medication or other forms of healing). These narrative resources of self-improvement and self-driven success can be useful and help women move through, survive and construct a sense of self that has the capacity to change and the power to do so.

This self-evaluative structure, shaped by an individualising and psychotherapeutic way of making sense of distress, can be useful, but it also functions to decontextualise people's struggles and distress. For example, Emma's quest to understand whether her distress was because of ADHD or 'all the trauma' points to an effort to find a 'neat' and coherent narrative that has logic and, therefore, renders her story readable to those she shares it with. However, it does not necessarily make space for the unique and complex ways that all aspects of her context and life experience intersect or even for both perspectives to be held as true.

Self-work and the quest for authenticity

This section of the chapter explores how participants I interviewed spoke about recoveries after domestic violence and, particularly, how a quest for authenticity was narrated as a key part of 'self-work'. When analysing participants' accounts, I noticed that some participants acknowledged that there can be a narrative disconnect between the past and present and that this narrative disconnect can bring about a sense of lacking authenticity. At the same time, in this conversation about authenticity, there was the assumption that living authentically is desired and synonymous with doing adulthood 'successfully' after adversities in childhood.

In Chapter 5, I explored how Liv spoke about the 'black mark' her childhood left her with and her struggles in young adulthood to navigate intimate partner relationships while bearing the mark and legacy of domestic violence in childhood. In this section of the chapter, I return to some of the interview with Liv. Liv was tearful in her interview as she spoke about difficulties with her mental health and the challenges in her relationship with her mother due to her being a carer for her mother, who was now disabled, and she described her as an alcoholic. As discussed in Chapter 5, she also described how she experiences 'problems' in relationships with men, which she attributed to the fact her father was violent. When talking about her mental health, she told her story in a way that centralised a drive and desire for things to be better:

> yeah I've been quite depressed the past couple of years. I was a lot more focused compared to how I am now, but I don't want just to resign myself to how I am now. I want to put plans in place because I know I'm not always gonna feel this way, or I hope I'm not
>
> *(Liv)*

Liv's account of the future was shaped by a voice of hope and a belief that things can be different. She said, 'I want to put plans in place... I know I'm not always gonna feel this way... I hope I'm not'. However, her voice of hope was constrained by the way that her difficulties immediately challenged the belief that things could change. The voice poem I constructed from the above interview extract demonstrates the I positions Liv spoke from:

> *I don't want just to resign myself to how I am now*
> *I want to put plans in place*
> *I know I'm not always gonna feel this way*
> *I hope I'm not*

The voice poem I constructed shows 'I as motivated to put work in and make plans for things to change' and 'I as hesitant'. When talking about the possibility of things getting better, one voice articulated a subtle hope. There is also perhaps an underlying doubt, which presses back against the voice of knowledge that things might – or perhaps even will – get better. This dialogue of voices produces tension in Liv's account that shows something about the challenge of telling a consistent story of the future when there also exists voices of doubt and uncertainty.

Voicing hope partly provided Liv with a sense of agency over her future story and self. The below extract from the interview shows Liv and I discussing her ideas about the future further:

Liv: *I feel like people can see – I feel like I wear my childhood on me. I feel like people think I'm a weirdo and stuff, and yeah. It puts me off like, mixing with people really*

Int: *yeah [pause] in like – in an ideal world now, can you tell me how things would be for you?*

Liv: erm, I think I would have pursued this career – but I struggled cos people said oh if you wanna get anywhere you're going to have to make contacts. And I was like oh, I'm never gonna make any contacts. You know? I didn't pursue it, but yeah I'd have like a partner and I'd be more financially stable. I think I used to be really good with finances and stuff but now I've kind of fallen into the same trap as my mum and I'm just terrified that I'm gonna end up [pause]

Int: it feels like you're in a trap? Like for you the same trap as your mum?

Liv: yeah, kind of like she's a black hole and I'm being dragged into it

Int: do you know what's dragging you into it?

Liv: just the way I've been brought up and it feels like I hit a load of blocks all the time. Even with jobs and stuff and you've got to be outgoing and I just feel like [sighs]

Int: it's not always easy to keep up with all of that

Liv: no

Int: it's not easy. No – I guess I'm struck with your feeling that you're being pulled into a black hole

Liv: It all weighs heavy on you. Like [pause] it's actually really hard to describe, but I feel like others can see it and I feel like it makes me different. And I feel like it's like a tie – that I'm gonna end up like that. I do pick bad relationships and stuff – and I don't even notice I'm doing it sometimes.

Through her account, despite the tie of the 'black hole', the visibility of her differences and trauma of her childhood, Liv's future self can be different. She said, 'I'd have a partner, I'd be more financially stable'. An alternative story acts as a counter-voice and counter-story to the shame that is associated with her childhood (Bamberg & Andrews, 2004). Being invited to consider alternative versions of her future enabled her to imagine the possibility of a different story. However, alternative stories have limited ways of being told and that is in part due to the dominance of narrative frameworks of risk and inevitable damage. The dominance of a risk and damage narrative resource can be seen through Liv's statement, 'she's a black hole and I'm being dragged into it'. It is also assumed that falling into that trap is something that Liv herself would be responsible for, as explored in Chapter 5. Jo Woodiwiss (2014), through her work exploring women's accounts of childhood sexual abuse, has suggested that in the absence of 'successful' healing and recovery stories, women who have experienced childhood trauma and abuse can fall back to a story of self-blame by claiming responsibility for their difficulties and by storying their adult difficulties as a direct consequence of their childhood trauma. While Liv's hope and belief that the future can be different is not entirely unspeakable or silenced, it is consistently knocked back through the existence of an individualising narrative framework that positions women themselves as responsible for their own self-making and self-healing after trauma. From this view, Liv storied her future self with uncertainty and tension, with self-blame and doubt threading through stories of potential futures.

Like Liv, Sonia also narrated her transition to young adulthood and her desire to make positive changes in her adult life. Sonia had grown up in a small rural part of England, and for most of her childhood, she experienced her father's physical and emotional violence towards her mother. Sonia explained how difficult it was to live in such a rural location where everybody knew everybody's lives. Yet somehow, it felt like nobody did anything about her father's very loud and obvious violence. She explained that as a teenager, she wanted everyone to think that she was 'from a normal family'. However, now, she felt very differently, and she no longer wanted to live with a 'mask' on:

> it's quite strange because now I'm more honest as an adult and [pause] yeah, I just feel like if I carry on living like this, it's almost like you know, you're living with a mask on I suppose. But it just caused me so much stress. So now I'd just really rather be open and honest. Not about what happened in detail, it's only really my partner that knows about that side, but I try and kind of say to people "oh I didn't really have a good relationship with my parents". So I'm more open to saying things like that now, so the more I've said it, I often receive the same reaction, which is shock. Erm, and I don't know if that's because people think, oh you know, she's got a professional job or I don't know
>
> *(Sonia)*

Central to Sonia's account is a drive and desire to live more authentically and no longer feel a need to conceal parts of her life that have perhaps carried shame in the past. She discusses the importance of making parts of her life more speakable in order to live more authentically and carry less stress. Through her account, becoming an adult and occupying a new identity, 'I as professional' meant that Sonia was, in part, no longer concerned about being 'normal' and 'fitting in' (something that is linked to childhood). As such, adulthood was an opportunity to re-story the self as 'successful', and it was an opportunity to live in an open way that causes her 'less stress'. However, 'I as professional' does not always align with her desire for honesty and authenticity in the face of others who may assume a professional with a job cannot also have experienced struggle. The below voice poem brings to light some of the intersecting voices that shaped her account of navigating young adulthood and authenticity.

I'm more honest as an adult
I just feel like if I carry on living like this –

you're living with a mask on
I'd just really rather be open and honest.
I try and kind of say
I didn't really have a good relationship with my parents
I'm more open to saying things like that
(people think)… she's got a professional job
I don't know

The voice poem shows the interplay between voices in Sonia's account. There is a voice of shame, 'you're living with a mask on', and there also exists a co-existing wish to be authentic, 'I'd just really rather be open and honest'. The dialogue between shame and a desire to be authentic is shaped by a story that positions openness and authenticity as ideal. There is a sense that while she lives with a mask on, and has done for most of her life, the mask is unwanted; it has implications and is no longer worth the stress.

On the one hand, authenticity was storied as ideal living, but the desire for authenticity was not the only voice in Sonia's account. In some contexts, Sonia's position as a successful adult professional can constrain how she can voice her struggles, increasing the weight of shame despite a desire to be open. The part of herself that wanted to be open and honest – the part of her that did not want to 'carry on living like this… living with a mask on', was restricted by the social narrative resources that imply that, particularly for women, being successful professionally does not allow space for personal struggle (Chowdhury et al., 2020).

In my interview with Hayley, in narrating her recovery process, she also centred a quest to live more authentically. Hayley had experienced substantial and multiple forms of violence and abuse in her childhood. She experienced her mother directing her father's violence towards her and her siblings, and she also experienced parental domestic abuse whereby both parents were physically violent towards each other. She described that for most of her adolescence, she had struggled with mental illness relating to an eating disorder and trauma. She also explained, during the interview, that she is now very open about her experiences and attributed her openness to the fact that she is now a therapist and that she only surrounds herself with those who are willing to hear her:

> I talk about my experiences a lot – it's part of my way of coping with my life presently. It's like how do I fit into normal society? Because if people talk about their childhood or whatever, it's like 'oh I don't have that experience' and I went through a period of just being quiet – like, just don't say it cos people will judge you, whereas now I keep people in my life that would let me say it and wouldn't judge me – they might still occasionally be shocked and fall off their chair or cry, which is always

really awkward – like you know it's sad, like my therapist brain knows it is sad but like my emotional response isn't necessarily appropriate. Erm and I keep those people in my life now – that are willing to hear it. Which means it's almost become quite normal for me to talk about it. It doesn't particularly bother me to talk about it. I don't very often like stop and take stock of how much things have changed.

(Hayley)

Hayley pointed to a time when she did not speak about her experiences because of the judgement of others. She pointed out, 'I went through a period of being quiet – like, just don't say it cos people will judge you, whereas now I keep people in my life that would let me say it and wouldn't judge me'. The capacity for openness and authenticity was storied as a process, something that Hayley had taken action to achieve and something that she had worked hard at. She reflected, 'I keep those people in my life now – that are willing to hear it'. From this view, the transition to openness and authenticity was storied as work, and it is storied as something that is a desirable and central part of this recovery story. I statements such as 'I talk about my experiences a lot…' and 'it's quite normal for me to talk about it. It doesn't particularly bother me to talk about it' write the self into a position of openness and authenticity, positioning the self as having done self-development work successfully. A recovery story of self-development and authenticity can be useful as it can support the production of a coherent self with a consistent and clear narrative of transition through which the past is narratively connected to the present.

This self-development narrative resource also underpins some of Emma's account. As I began to explore earlier in this chapter, Emma's account evidenced multiple voices, which suggested a grappling with a self-pathologising voice, a quest to know and understand her struggles and a voice of self-compassion. I understand these voices as efforts to story the self through a self-development narrative resource in a context whereby authenticity and self-work are valuable, particularly for women who have experienced trauma and are navigating recovery. Emma explained that it was only since she started studying psychology that she had begun to figure herself out and realise what was 'right':

I felt awful… I was just like, this is not right… I think I'm only, in the last four years, starting to figure myself out… I think my course has saved my life really

(Emma)

Through Emma's account, she positioned self-knowledge and self-development as having the capacity to be transformative, to the extent that studying psychology as a way of better understanding herself had saved her life. It also positioned self-development as crucial to her ability to tell a different story where she is different from her mother. Stories of ongoing learning and transition were made possible through the new identity positions that Emma occupied as an adult and as a student of psychology. These new identity positions enabled stories of change that, in part, were useful recovery stories to tell.

The way that Emma explained, 'I'm only, in the last four years, starting to figure myself out', points to the ongoing voice of self-development and the work of recovery, according to this way of storying recovery. The fact that she is 'only starting' implies that there is more to go and that the development story has not ended. Drawing on Dialogical Self Theory (Hermans, 2003, 2022), this ongoing quality draws attention to the unfinalisability of the narrative self and points to the way that Emma's story challenges the idea that a developmental transition from childhood to adulthood, as it intersects with recovery after childhood domestic violence, is one where there is an endpoint.

Resilience and choosing the 'better life'

As well as self-development stories and stories that were centred around a quest for authenticity, recovery stories included accounts of resilience, choosing a better life and finding ways to move on. Storying recovery by centring resilience and individual choice and autonomy enabled women to write themselves into a different kind of life than the one that they had experienced in childhood. At the same time, these stories were limiting as they restricted space to voice emotion, particularly emotion that might destabilise a coherent and credible recovery story and 'survivor' identity.

Frances was a university student when we met for the interview. She had grown up in a city and had experienced the traumatic loss of a sibling when she was very young, as well as physical and emotional abuse directed towards her from both her parents and parental domestic abuse perpetrated by both parents towards each other. She described several efforts to tell teachers at school and even to tell social workers about what was happening, but none believed her. She also disclosed to a social worker about the violence, and she was not believed this time either. Frances described struggling with a severe eating disorder in her late teens and a sense that she did not know how she stayed alive or kept on going. She found that studying was something she was good at, and she described a huge motivation to get herself into good schools and to university. A central part of Frances' recovery story was her pride that she had chosen the 'better life' and shown resilience in doing so:

> it just kind of shines a light to me about how resilient I am and how proud I am of myself. But then talking about it, and reflecting on it with you,

has started like a bit of an anger fireball going, where I just think how did I get let down so badly? How did I get ignored by the people that could have got me out of that situation so many times? And it makes me feel sad for other people that may have experienced similar things to me but they didn't have the resilience to choose the better life. And they would have just been let down by all these people and by the system... Erm you know, potentially revisiting kind of like the social services that let me down is something that I have thought about, you know... But for me to do that I need to know that – I need to be ready to do that, and right now I'm not ready to do that

(Frances)

Frances' account foregrounded a story of pride and resilience. However, a voice of anger also exists that does not always align with a stable and credible account of resilience.

I would never want anyone to experience what I went through or the feelings that I had to endure or the behaviour that I was subjected to. I'd never want anyone to go through that. And the way I could do it is by going back to the services and giving them some feedback. But then on the flipside I just think, well what's the point? They let me down before, they're not gonna take my feedback seriously. And that trust isn't there. And that almost kind of – on their part I don't want to cooperate with them because I'm angry with them, but then I want to be able to help others. So it's just kind of this thing that I need to navigate.

(Frances)

Frances highlighted her sense of resilience and suggested one of the reasons for her participating in my research was that she did not want others to experience the same. Using her experience for good in order to help others is framed as central to a recovery story in which she has chosen 'the better life'. However, a story of resilience and recovery is at odds with the anger that is also voiced. I constructed the following voice poem from the above extract from the interview. In the voice poem, I have included the 'I' and I have also included 'They', where Frances talks about 'They' as the services that let her down:

I just think, well what's the point?
They let me down before
they're not gonna take my feedback seriously
I don't want to cooperate with them
I'm angry with them
I want to be able to help others

The voice poem demonstrates the interplay between 'I as resilient' (voiced through a story of wanting to help others), 'I as angry and let down' (voiced as a part that is angry at services and does not want to cooperate) and 'I as hopeless' (voiced through a story of 'what's the point?'). The voice poem, as I see it, helps to show how these voices exist in dialogue with one another. The way I read it is that, in a way, anger is a voice that becomes less speakable, existing on the margins or becoming silenced in favour of an account of resilience. This resilience enables space for a certain version of recovery – 'I want to help others' and 'I chose the better life', but this version is compromised by 'I as angry' and 'I as hopeless'; parts that are not ready or that maybe do not see any point because her anger is *too* much.

In examining the dialogical relationship between voices here, there is a sense that Frances did not feel she could put her anger to use because she was *too* angry – she was not ready and did not see the point. Anger is storied as raw emotion, unprocessed and as producing a sense of incoherency. Thinking more broadly about emotion in recovery stories – anger in this case – can be understood by drawing on Sara Ahmed's (2014) theorisations of emotion as both individual and politically and socially constituted, produced and expressed. Frances' account that she was 'too angry' to speak points to the power at play in the socio-cultural context that shaped how she told her story. Using her experience to do good by speaking out and helping others is part of a neoliberal recovery story of individual strength and success, and this kind of story allowed her to talk about gaining strength and empowerment. However, Frances' recovery story is, at the same time, shaped by neoliberal ideologies that risk silencing the anger she carries – so much so that she concludes, 'It's just kind of this thing I need to navigate'. Anger is also storied in the context of a history where her account has been discredited and she has not been believed. This is testimonial injustice, a form of epistemic injustice whereby a speaker's marginalised social positioning means they are less likely to be seen and heard as a credible narrator. Frances' social positioning as a child, and perhaps also as a girl, contributed to the epistemic injustice she experienced, which drives the voice of anger now.

I make sense of this anger and testimonial injustice as operating within gendered power relations. In the context of survival after trauma, if women speak with 'too much' emotion, then it is said to 'transgress appropriate survivor talk', leading women to police themselves and be policed in relation to their emotions (Alcoff & Gray, 1993, p. 285). Frances' anger at the way she had been let down by services motivated her to consider going back to services to give them feedback in the hopes it would help others. Frances also voiced ambivalence about how her anger can be expressed and how it may be heard and read by others. Women can have particular ambivalence about how anger is expressed and used because anger is not always considered synonymous with femininity (Holmes, 2004).

Others have suggested that women expressing anger on their own behalf can function to pose a threat to a patriarchal society where women are generally invited to stay small, and anger is typically seen as a masculine expression (Alcoff & Gray, 1993). Thus, through a neoliberal recovery story, women might be more able to express anger on behalf of others, as expressing anger on behalf of others rather than on behalf of the self is a more 'appropriate' and acceptable response to violence, and it is more likely to be read and heard as a recognisable and credible story of recovery. Considered in this way, Frances' proposal to go back to services so that the same does not happen to others is central to her recovery story. It functions to stabilise a story that may be destabilised by expressing anger on behalf of herself.

These narrative resources of credibility, femininity and emotion also intersect with Frances' sense of pride that she chose the 'better life' and had the resilience to do so. Some participants spoke about being OK enough to tell their stories – about having done the work to enable them to feel OK with talking openly about their experiences. Others said the interview was the first time that they had spoken openly about their experiences, but they felt a responsibility to contribute to research to help others. Regardless of how participants framed their capacity and motivation to share their stories, a sense of having moved through to the other side, a sense of having 'travelled through', puts their struggles in the past and supports the narrative construction of the self as being self-knowledgeable and having survived. A survival position is not explicitly named as 'survivor' in participants' accounts, but the way that participants narrated recovery, resilience, self-development and 'travelling through', from my reading, does seem to align in some way with dominant discourses that surround survivorship (Alcoff & Gray, 1993; Orgad, 2009; Ovenden, 2012). Survival stories such as these can be both empowering and limiting. They can provide a framework for talking about trauma and recovery in a way that others can hear, and they can help construct the self as resilient. However, stories that construct 'I as survivor' can simultaneously be limiting (Alcoff & Gray, 1993; Reich, 2002); struggles can be difficult to articulate because of the lack of favourable and supportive narrative frameworks through which to tell them.

Forgiving, forgetting and moving on

Recovery stories were also shaped by the self-development work required to use inner strength and 'move on'. I now want to think about my interview with Jasmine. I introduced Jasmine in Chapter 5, where I explored briefly the way in which she storied her memories of her father's anger and violence being used as a tool not to become angry or violent herself. In my interview with Jasmine, she spoke about gaining strength from her experiences. She explained:

> in order to forget I've kind of gotta forgive what happened… forgive what I was put through and accept that it was part of life… that did happen to me but it doesn't necessarily mean that my whole life has to be ruined.
>
> *(Jasmine)*

Central to Jasmine's account was a story of the self-development work she had done to forgive, forget and move on. These stories of healing, strength and forgiveness functioned to establish her as no longer impacted by the violence she grew up with. I asked Jasmine what it was like to reflect on her childhood. She responded:

> Because I have dealt with it, it always feels like I'm talking about someone else, which is really weird.] It's just something that I think, because I'm so at peace with it now, it's just something that kind of happened, like I brushed my teeth yesterday, like I brushed my teeth this morning. It's just something that happened that is just [pause] part of who I am
>
> *(Jasmine)*

Her account of moving on functioned to establish a sense of narrative distance, positioning childhood as something she is no longer impacted by; it is just 'something that happened':

> when I'm talking about it I picture myself as a little girl, and that's who I'm talking about. And obviously I know that I am that little girl, but it's kind of like all of that happened to a little girl and that isn't me. Although it is – but it's just like I've lived like two lives
>
> *(Jasmine)*

I want to show the voice poem I created from the above interview extract to explore a little more of the multiple I positions in Jasmine's account. In the voice poem, I have also included two lines that indicate the 'I' but where the 'I' has dropped off and is not used:

> *I picture myself as a little girl… that's who I'm talking about*
> *I know*
> *I am that little girl*
> *that isn't me*
> *Although it is*
> *I've lived like two lives*

This gap between experiencing ('it's kind of like all that happened to a little girl and that isn't me') and knowledge ('I know I am that little girl') is something that Hydén (2014) notes is common for people who have previously been victimised. She suggests that telling stories that help to establish a sense of distance can be a form of psychological protection against overwhelming pain. A sense of distance can be understood as having a narrative function that does something useful for Jasmine by establishing a sense of psychological safety. However, distance and disconnect do not align well with the autobiographical coherence and connectedness of the therapeutic recovered self that requires a story that can connect the past to the present in a linear and coherent way. At the same time, this distance helps to position Jasmine as secure in her adult identity and affords her epistemic privilege. In this position, she is more likely to be considered a trustworthy source of knowledge, bolstering the strength and wisdom that her recovery story writes her into. She reflected:

> I think I'm definitely stronger, wiser – erm, but I still have inner conflicts about that because I sometimes wanna be that little girl again
>
> *(Jasmine)*

Jasmine's acknowledgement of these conflicts suggests there is a challenge in narrating a childhood that her adult self does not identify with, yet which she knows was part of her life. Jasmine's articulation, 'I know I am that little girl', but 'that little girl isn't me', followed by the knowledge that 'it is' her illustrates this tussle and suggests that recovery, rather than being linear, could be considered fluid, dynamic and perhaps even interrupted or fragmented in places. Jasmine reflected that she had 'dealt with her demons', but her conflicting feelings were not entirely left in her childhood:

> It's all confusing, I think. I just don't know how people – I do know how you process it, like I said, I think the biggest way to get over something is to forgive that it happened. I think if you don't forgive that it happened, it's always going to be a demon in the back of your mind if that makes sense
>
> *(Jasmine)*

Through this account, Jasmine has put her 'demons' behind her, and at the same time, she still might find it confusing to process or make sense of. This hesitancy serves to break that sense of narrative distance. It suggests that recovery is not as simple as 'moving on', but it is fluid, dynamic and consists of conflicts that may get erased through linear stories that do not account for fluidity and interchanging positions.

Summary

This chapter has explored how women's recovery stories consisted of multiple stories: stories that draw on psychotherapeutic self-evaluative narrative frameworks, stories that centre a quest for authenticity and stories that centre the self-work required to acquire individual resilience and a 'better life'. In this chapter, I have shown that while dominant assumptions about recovery after domestic violence – and more broadly, after trauma – are that recovery is linear and has an endpoint, this does not always align with how participants told their stories. This chapter has explored how dominant foregrounded voices exist in dialogue with the more marginalised and difficult-to-articulate voices, including voices of 'excess' 'uncontainable' emotion, struggle and uncertainty.

Participants had not accessed services or received support to address their experiences of domestic violence. Given that their childhood experiences of domestic violence took place out of the gaze of services or institutions that might have validated and legitimised their experiences, there are limited ways of talking about it or even naming it as domestic violence. Previous research has explored the power of an authorised account of domestic violence, suggesting that professionalised or therapeutic discourses can shape childhood accounts, as these accounts are readable and accepted versions of the violence that happened (Callaghan et al., 2017). This chapter has shown that these authorised accounts do not always fit with lived experiences of abuse, and they serve to smoothen out the multivocality of the expression of their experiences. However, authorised accounts also can provide a stable story that is more likely to be considered reliable by those listening.

This chapter examines how power plays a significant part in shaping recovery stories, as gendered social structures operate in ways that can be both limiting and empowering. Neoliberal values of self-improvement and self-responsibility pave the way for what kind of recoveries are possible to talk about, and this intersects with gender in important ways. For example, telling a recovery story that does not contain 'too much' emotion or struggle is useful; it can provide a quality of coherency that has the capacity to stabilise the therapeutic recovered self. However, this risks women self-narrating stories in which they alone are responsible for their happiness and recovery, erasing the social, relational and political ways in which recovery and violence are located (Rose, 2010; Wastell & White, 2012). I have explored that individualising psychotherapeutic narrative frameworks can function to invite all adulthood difficulties to be correlated with the abuse experienced in childhood, and this can limit the way that recovery stories can be articulated. Feminist scholars have argued that contemporary northern narrative frameworks locate femininities or womanhood within individualising discourses of self-work and self-improvement (Gill & Scharff, 2011; McRobbie, 2004).

As such, neoliberal values surround a particular kind of femininity whereby a successful and speakable recovery is self-made and self-driven. This chapter concludes that dominant recovery narrative frameworks do something useful for participants in providing a coherent story, but they also put significant limitations on what kind of story of recovery is possible to tell.

References

Ahmed, S. (2014). *The cultural politics of emotion* (2nd ed.). Edinburgh University Press.

Alcoff, L., & Gray, L. (1993). Survivor discourse: Transgression or recuperation? *Signs: Journal of Women in Culture and Society, 18*(2), 260–290. https://doi.org/10.1086/494793

Bamberg, M., & Andrews, M. (2004). *Considering counter narratives: Narrating, resisting, making sense.* John Benjamins Publishing Company.

Callaghan, J. E. M., Fellin, L. C., Mavrou, S., Alexander, J., & Sixsmith, J. (2017). The management of disclosure in children's accounts of domestic violence: Practices of telling and not telling. *Journal of Child and Family Studies, 26*(12), 3370–3387. https://doi.org/10.1007/s10826-017-0832-3

Chowdhury, N., Gibson, K., & Wetherell, M. (2020). Polyphonies of depression: The relationship between voices-of-the-self in young professional women aka "top girls." *Health, 24*(5), 773–790. https://doi.org/10.1177/1363459319846934

Gill, R., & Scharff, C. (2011). *New femininities: Postfeminism, neoliberalism, and subjectivity.* Palgrave Macmillan.

Hermans, H. J. M. (2003). The construction and reconstruction of a dialogical self. *Journal of Constructivist Psychology, 16*(2), 89–130. https://doi.org/10.1080/10720530390117902

Hermans, H. J. M. (2022). *Liberation in the face of uncertainty. A new development in dialogical self theory.* Cambridge University Press.

Holmes, M. (2004). Feeling beyond rules: Politicizing the sociology of emotion and anger in feminist politics. *European Journal of Social Theory, 7*(2), 209–227. https://doi.org/10.1177/1368431004041752

Hydén, M. (2014). The teller-focused interview: Interviewing as a relational practice. *Qualitative Social Work: Research and Practice, 13*(6), 795–812. https://doi.org/10.1177/1473325013506247

McRobbie, A. (2004). Post-feminism and popular culture. *Feminist Media Studies, 4*(3), 255–264. https://doi.org/10.1080/1468077042000309937

Orgad, S. (2009). The survivor in contemporary culture and public discourse: A genealogy. *The Communication Review, 12*(2), 132–161. https://doi.org/10.1080/10714420902921168

Ovenden, G. (2012). Young women's management of victim and survivor identities. *Culture, Health & Sexuality, 14*(8), 941–954. https://doi.org/10.1080/13691058.2012.710762

Reich, N. M. (2002). Towards a rearticulation of women-as-victims: A thematic analysis of the construction of women's identities surrounding gendered violence. *Communication Quarterly, 50*(3–4), 292–311. https://doi.org/10.1080/01463370209385665

Rose, N. (1985). *The psychological complex: Psychology, politics, and society in England, 1869–1939*. Routledge & Kegan Paul.

Rose, N. (2010). 'Screen and intervene': Governing risky brains. *History of the Human Sciences, 23*(1), 79–105. https://doi.org/10.1177/0952695109352415

Wastell, D., & White, S. (2012). Blinded by neuroscience: Social policy, the family and the infant brain. *Families, Relationships and Societies, 1*(3), 397–414. https://doi.org/10.1332/204674312X656301

Woodiwiss, J. (2014). Beyond a single story: The importance of separating 'harm' from 'wrongfulness' and 'sexual innocence' from 'childhood' in contemporary narratives of childhood sexual abuse. *Sexualities, 17*(1–2), 139–158. https://doi.org/10.1177/1363460713511104

7
PRECARIOUS WORK AND CREATIVE ASSEMBLAGES OF VOICE/S

I know from a rational point of view it's just crazy
 I know him
 I love him
I thought no
I've had such a lot of conflict about it
            ~ Voice poem created from the interview with Bethany

Introduction

In narrative psychology, life story coherence is related to psychological well-being (Baerger & McAdams, 1999). Additionally, trauma literature understands an integrated and coherent life story is often one of the aims of trauma therapy (Herman, 2015). As explored in the previous two chapters, young women's accounts of transitions and recoveries consisted of multiple-voiced storylines. Sometimes, these voices can be understood as contrapuntal voices, meaning there were tensions and contradictions between storylines and between voiced accounts.

Because these kinds of inner conflicts were so central to women's accounts, I became interested in the creative strategies women used to resist being read as not credible and unreliable self-narrators as they told stories of survival through and after trauma and violence. This is what I mean when I write about precarious work. I see some of the creative strategies as complex, precarious narrative strategies that women used in efforts to reject individualising hegemonic discourses about survival and recovery, which did not serve them well. At the same time, women re-inscribed these narrative resources in

DOI: 10.4324/9781003393160-7

instances where they partially served them well. This chapter is an exploration of these creative narrative strategies. According to the Cambridge Dictionary (2024), 'Precarious' means 'in a dangerous state because of not being safe or not being held in place firmly'. I consider these strategies as precarious work because these strategies get used precisely when marginalised or less-dominant stories are voiced. These are stories that may be considered dangerous or unsafe to voice in some contexts . They are stories where the 'I' is not stable, and articulating this instability becomes risky.

Chess and black holes: storying tensions and contradictions through metaphor

In Chapter 6, I discussed how participants drew on dominant narrative frameworks of survival when they spoke about recovery from domestic violence in childhood. Not only was survival framed through recovery stories as a desired outcome, but also survival was storied as a non-linear path despite the dominance of recovery narrative frameworks that are linear and offer more epistemic power as they are more likely to be read and heard as legible and credible stories. In this section, I build on these arguments by exploring how women storied survival as ambiguous, ongoing and tensioned.

In Chapter 5, I explored Clara's 'growing up' story, where she spoke about a sudden realisation that suddenly, she was a grown-up and needed to cope with the impacts of her father's violence while she was still a young child. Clara also spoke about the impact of her father continuing the abuse through the courts.

> Often the court cases and stuff are between mum, [sibling] and my dad. Because he still pays maintenance for [sibling]. And I'm often disregarded, and that's fine, you know, I don't mind not being part of it. But when there is an impact on me, I want them to be brought up because I think it's important they get a picture of what's going on. If they go to court and the judge doesn't know that I've been told to sell my car or that I've been missed off a form, you know, I'm just totally ignored. Or he's said something nasty to me in a letter or directed something at me, and that's not said… how is the judge ever gonna get a picture of this man, he's just gonna see what the solicitors want him to see.
>
> *(Clara)*

Clara was involved in legal proceedings because she was also a carer for her sibling, who had additional needs. She explained that court proceedings happened regularly each time her dad withheld maintenance money. She was often excluded from the court proceedings, and this meant the judge did not get a full picture of her dad's abuse and its impact. Given that the court proceedings were ongoing, survival was not something that Clara spoke about retrospectively, but it was ongoing. From one voice, Clara wanted to be included in the court proceedings, and she wanted the things that her dad did that impacted her, such as writing nasty letters and withholding money, to be accounted for in court. It bothered her that she was excluded. However, she also said, 'I'm often disregarded, and that's fine, you know, I don't mind not being a part of it'. Clara occupied two seemingly incongruous positions about her involvement in the court proceedings. I consider this as a tension that may have been challenging to articulate coherently. To articulate the contradictory voices, she used metaphor as a way of inviting me to hear:

Clara: *there's a lot of stuff going on, a lot of power dynamics and a lot of control dynamics. I think everybody has a role and everybody has a place in it. It's almost like a game of chess. My mum calls it that actually*
Int: *Game of chess?*
Clara: *yeah she says it's a game of chess – I've always got to be one move ahead otherwise he'll get me*

Using chess as a metaphor enabled Clara to communicate something about the complexities of negotiating power and place within the family:

Clara: *dad probably likes to think that he's moving us, but he's not. Definitely not. But [sigh] I don't know where I'd put myself on a chess board with it. I'd like to think I'm not even on the chess board anymore, I mean I probably am because I'm still involved, but I'd like to be [drops off...]*
Int: *Where are you instead? Do you know where you'd like to be?*
Clara: *Like around the chess board. Just somewhere else [laughs]. I don't even care where, as long as I'm not playing the game, I don't really care. Like I can be my mum's cheerleader, you know what I mean? But I don't wanna be on the board, I don't wanna be involved.*

The voice poem shows some of the contradictory voices:

I'd like to think I'm not even on the chessboard
I mean
I probably am
I'm still involved
I'd like to be...
I don't even care where

I don't really care.
I can be my mum's cheerleader
I don't wanna be on the board
I don't wanna be involved.

This story is voiced through 'I as not caring and not wanting to be involved', alongside 'I as mother's cheerleader and still in the game'. Clearly, one cannot be both a cheerleader and uninvolved completely. However, the use of the chess game as a metaphor was a way of inviting me to stay with the hesitancy and contradiction. Her account suggests that she did not want to be involved in these games, yet her very existence in her family relationships means that she is. The tension here is narrated through this metaphor as a constant to and fro, a desire to be both in the game and out of it. Clara felt strongly about the times when she was overlooked in court proceedings, even though her father's ongoing abuse and coercive control still impacted her. Clara's statements, 'I don't care… I don't wanna be on the board, I don't wanna be involved', suggest a voice of struggle that is constrained and simultaneously a voice of self-sufficient survival that has power.

The risk of storying the self as still involved and emotionally impacted is that Clara may write herself into a position of helplessness or lacking autonomy in her survival. There are limited narrative resources that provide a useful framework through which Clara could talk about her experience of surviving the abuse and coercive control her dad continued to use towards Clara, her mother and her sibling. In Chapter 6, I discussed that dominant discourses surrounding survival from violence or abuse are typically framed through neoliberal ideologies (Beck & Beck-Gernsheim, 2002; Rose, 1992, 2010), and these can shape storytelling practices about recovery and survival. I explored that telling a survival story carries social, cultural and political power because it can provide coherency. The power of these survival narrative resources significantly constrains the speakability of other voices. From this view, to tell a survival story that is logical and stable, she needs not to care in order to survive. However, the need to not care constrains the speakability of the voices that do care, the parts that are still involved and the parts that might experience tensions or struggle.

Clara's storytelling practices evidence the challenges that arise when dominant narrative frameworks fail young women. McKenzie-Mohr and Lafrance (2011) wrote about the use of metaphor as a strategy to help women talk about the nuances of their experiences when dominant narrative resources fail them. In Clara's account, the metaphor of a chess game functioned as a strategy for her to communicate contradictions and negotiate power. It also suggests that the 'game' is not an individual game; chess is a fluid and dynamic game. When one person moves, so does the other, and there are opportunities for negotiation and movement.

In Chapter 5, I also introduced Nadine, who had experienced serious and severe physical and sexual violence from her father, including violence towards herself. In Chapter 5, I explored how Nadine navigated transitions to young adulthood in the face of mental health professionals telling her she should not have children in case she turned out violent like her father. Like Clara, Nadine also used metaphor to articulate tensions and contradictions:

> if I didn't come to university, I don't know what I would have done with my life. It's just that [Int: yeah] and that feels like a hole – like a really big black hole that you just fall down into there, if you didn't have to keep going, you'd think too much
>
> *(Nadine)*

The metaphor of a 'black hole' evidences a voice of fear that she would fall into a black hole if she did not have something to keep her going. This metaphor captures the need to hold on to something to keep her from falling. Like the chess metaphor, the black hole metaphor is a useful strategy. Phrases such as 'you just fall down into there' enable Nadine to communicate a story of despair, assuming a sense of inevitability. At the same time, a voice of strength, that 'you have to keep going', despite the gravitational pull of the 'black hole', bolsters a thread of agency and strength. Existing narrative resources about women's success and survivorship do not make space for co-existing stories of struggle and despair that were voiced through the black hole metaphor.

Gendered social structures and individualising ideologies shape how this metaphor was used. Dominant narrative resources that are available to women in Western contexts are shaped around the idea that if women remain positive and productive even in the face of struggle and adversity, then they will eventually live happy and successful lives (Chowdhury, Gibson, & Wetherell, 2020; Gill & Orgad, 2018; Gill & Scharff, 2011). The feminisation of success has been explored in the literature, which suggests that post-feminist discourses have reshaped womanhood around individualising ideologies in Western contexts (Adkins, 2001; Chowdhury et al., 2020; McRobbie, 2004, 2015). Instead of assumptions that women are passive and vulnerable, 'women are drawn on as a metaphor for social progress' (Baker, 2010, p. 2). However, the feminisation of success and increasing autonomy shapes the discursive landscape within which women told their stories. Nadine's emphasis on her efforts to keep going despite the struggle of resisting the gravitational pull of the black hole communicates that keeping on going in the face of the gravitational pull of the black hole is a battle. However, I understand this is also a story that enables her to write herself into a desirable position of having successfully done recovery work in the face of adversity.

Narrating survival as a battle

Narrating survival as a battle brings to light tensions and contradictions that may otherwise be overlooked. Framing survival as a battle in this way can be seen as a strategy for inviting the listener to hear the nuances of stories. Nadine spoke about her fight to stay at school:

> I tried to get help in that year saying that my mum's really ill and this is why I'm not coming into school, well, sixth form, and this is why my grades are slipping… nothing was done about it. It was just, I was seen as this problem. So I really had to fight to come back for the third year because they were saying 'well your attendance, you're not gonna come back, you're not gonna get these grades'. It was just mad
>
> *(Nadine)*

Nadine's emphasis on the need to fight to keep going demonstrates the function and use of this 'fight' or 'battle' story. It highlights the power of this story in a socio-cultural context that values self-made recovery stories, as discussed in Chapter 6. In some ways, storying survival as a fight enables women to demonstrate the agency and autonomy deemed necessary to occupy a successful position as young women. For example, Nadine said: 'I really had to fight to come back'. Clara also said: 'I've got my own life now', and as I discussed in Chapter 6, Frances reflected: 'I feel sad for other people that may have experienced similar things to me, but they didn't have the resilience to choose the better life'. Nadine's 'black hole' metaphor was used to communicate deep despair and distress and to recognise her agency and choice. It enabled her to both inscribe *and* resist neoliberal ideologies that shape dominant narrative frameworks of survivorship and success.

Frances had made several disclosures about the violence at home to adults and had not been believed. She spoke about her pride that despite everything, her strength and determination enabled her to keep going. When I asked Frances about what helped her to keep going, she fell to a place of not knowing:

> I honestly don't know, and I don't know how I ever picked myself up every single day and pretended that it wasn't happening. Like, I am not aware of how I did that
>
> *(Frances)*

> I just don't know how I did that'… 'I didn't cope. I don't know how – I thought I was going to die, I was ready to give up
>
> *(Frances)*

Frances' survival story draws on 'I who did not cope and was ready to give up' and 'I who picked myself up despite thinking I could not'. The dialogical interplay of these voices produces a story of a fight for survival. Storying survival as a fight is one way of demonstrating both I positions; survival as a fight shines light on the alternative stories that women have available to them to tell if they do not have readable survival stories that consistently tell a story of success. A fight story also makes space for despair and struggle while centring and valuing the self-driven determination to push through. Frances was not the only participant who negotiated finding a coherent and integrated way to story the self from the past to the present. She is not the only participant whose experiences were not reflected in available narrative resources about how one survives. For example, Sochi and Emma also did not or did not have a way of articulating know how they had survived:

> I don't really know how to describe it really. Cos as I say, it is literally just carrying on... I think not thinking about stuff, not talking about stuff and just acting like it didn't really happen
>
> *(Sochi)*

> I felt so lost before, but not knowing that I felt lost, it was just confusion and frustration and anxiety. It wasn't a pleasant place to be. I actually don't really know how I kind of plodded on
>
> *(Emma)*

The gap between experience and knowledge – a disconnection between the before and after – is not uncommon for people who have experienced violence and abuse (Alcoff, 2018; Herman, 2015; Hydén, 2014). However, the fact that there are limited words available to make sense of how women kept carrying on suggests that women can tell stories of survival and struggle, but there are limited ways of storying the 'how'. When I asked whether Frances could say more about how she carried on, she explained that she was 'done with fighting':

> I very much didn't want to be alive. Very much did not want to be there, did not want to be alive anymore. I tried, I tried, you know?
>
> *(Frances)*

Storying the 'how' of the fight was told though 'I who wanted to die' and 'I who tried to stay alive'. The voice poem shows these I positions:

> *I very much didn't want to be alive*
> *I tried*

I tried
You know?

Frances' fight story was told through occupying a both/and position that recognises her distress ('I didn't want to be alive') and her agency ('I tried'). Occupying a 'both/and' position like this has been suggested to be a strategy employed by participants when dominant narrative frameworks fail them, but when there is also an important story to tell (McKenzie-Mohr & Lafrance, 2011). It is a creative strategy, in some ways, of inviting me as the listener to stay with and dwell in this ambiguously storied survival, one which is told through both 'I as surviving' and 'I as wanting to die'.

Navigating ontological (in)security

This section of the chapter explores the precarious narrative work of telling stories of who we are when the world has become uncertain, and others' realities may not align with one's own sense of the self. The idea of ontological security is rooted in existential psychoanalytical thinking (Laing 1960/2010). Human geographers (Giddens, 1991) have adopted the concept, coining the term 'ontological security', referring to 'a psychological achievement that enables most people, most of the time, to take for granted – to trust – that our ordinary, everyday worlds are reliable and dependable' (Bondi, 2014, p. 332). As such, ontological insecurity refers to situations of stress, crisis or distress where those living in precarious positions have lost that taken-for-grantedness and trust that our everyday worlds and environments can and will remain stable. As such, our place in the world becomes destabilised and disrupted when our own realities are seemingly at odds with the realities of others. Ontological insecurity can, therefore, be understood as when one experiences or perceives a threat to our subjective sense of who we are (Laing, 1960/2010).

Through stories of hope and loss, participants evidenced the challenge of telling stories that others may not understand. In Chapter 5, I introduced Bethany and explored how she narrated transitions to motherhood when she felt lost and did not know how to parent due to not having female role models herself. Here, I want to explore how she narrated the tensions and contradictions in her account of maintaining contact with her father after her parents separated:

Bethany: *I kept in contact with my dad, well I tried to. He was a total shit about it actually he let me down a lot, even up until having my daughter, but I still tried to keep in contact with him, which is so hard to understand from the outside, you know. Why would you want to?*
Int: *can you tell me a bit about how you've tried to keep in contact with him and what that's been like for you?*

Bethany: oh well, when he, when he left my mum I think he did that whole thing of extending the abuse through child contact court. They went to court for ages and wrangled with the kids. Anyway they decided it would be once a month at a weekend, and I don't think my mum disclosed domestic violence to the court actually at the time anyway, so she was going through this thing, you know, without them realising that either. Because it just wasn't the done thing, well she didn't you know – never tell anyone. So he would just hardly ever turn up, so he spent all this time getting the order and then he would mess my mum around really or not turn up and then she'd have to meet him half way and she'd be in cold sweats like dripping, and most of the time I wasn't involved because it wasn't like I could decide.

Bethany articulated the challenges she faced when trying to maintain contact with her father and constantly being let down. Bethany had experienced being 'wrangled with' through the court and contact with her father was mandated post-separation. However, she had also chosen to try to maintain contact with her dad into adulthood. She reflected on the way that she was 'emotionally torn' and her account evidences the challenge of narrating a coherent story about why she wanted to maintain contact. I include the voice poem here that includes the 'he' and 'you' as a way of maintaining the context of the account and the way each voice tells a particular story:

I kept in contact with my dad
I tried to.
He was a total shit about it
he let me down a lot
I still tried to keep in contact with him
Why would you want to?
he would just hardly ever turn up
I wasn't involved
it wasn't like I could decide
he was just –
he just let you down

On the one hand, Bethany wanted contact with her father. There also exists a voice that questioned, 'why would you want to?'. The questioning voice is bolstered by the reality of what happened when she tried to meet up with her dad – the fact that she was let down constantly. Her wish for contact is constantly shut down because that wish for contact compromises the stability and consistency of the account. Bethany spoke more about this conflict:

> He told me that he was on his way and I waited for an hour with a new born and he didn't turn up and it's just constant. And I can't believe I never – this is the thing, in my professional life, I never tell anyone - oh god, I still gave him chances till I was 28. You know, he walked me down the aisle on my wedding day because I always felt like "well what if we made it up once and I regretted it?" – it's like that hope never goes, even though you totally, you can totally rationalise this person is bad. But you're brought up thinking that's my dad – and if I don't – if I don't, if I lose contact with him, I lose, that's my dad. It's so confusing and that's the problem with it all. It's very difficult for people to understand I think outside, especially feminist sort of women's organisations. They assume that you do not want contact with the perpetrator and I can't argue that's not absolutely the best thing most of the time, but as a child you don't feel like that – I mean I can't even say I'm a child in my 20's but literally my whole life, up until I became a mum it's like ok well that happened, and that's enough. You let me down again and that's enough, I never want to see you ever again, like
>
> *(Bethany)*

Bethany's account contained an orchestration of voices of rationality and emotion. A storyline of being 'emotionally torn' and confused was dominant. The voice poem shows the multiple subjectivities:

> *I can't believe I never –*
> *I never tell anyone –*
> *I still gave him chances till I was 28.*
> *he walked me down the aisle on my wedding day*
> *you can totally rationalise this person is bad.*
> *you're brought up thinking that's my dad –*
> *if I don't –*
> *if I don't,*
> *if I lose contact with him*
> *I lose, that's my dad.*
> *You let me down again and that's enough*
> *I never want to see you ever again*

Bethany's I position, 'I never want to see you again', exists in dialogue with voices of fear of loss. She explained that although she could no longer go through the pain of being let down, the cost of making a choice to cut contact also meant losing her dad. Her experience of her dad was one of constantly being let down, but her story is also powerfully shaped by narrative resources of idealised family life that offer Bethany hope but also constrain the articulation of the reality of her experiences of being hurt and let down. As such, the challenge of narrating 'I as let down' can be understood as ontological insecurity. The subjective reality of this voice is not reflected in the context in which she may often feel it or voice it. It is almost as if articulating this voice produces a sense of ontological insecurity that threatens the legibility and coherency of her account and herself. This ontological insecurity can be seen as a kind of hermeneutical injustice where parts of Bethany's knowledge and reality are seemingly difficult to communicate in an intelligible way to me as the listener or to 'anyone'. As such, this gap between hermeneutic resources produces an epistemic injustice that is shaped by a lack of shared tools of social interpretation. It is, in some ways, incomprehensible that she should want to keep her father in her life, after all the violence she endured from him. Yet at the same time, she makes efforts to communicate this tension. To negotiate this, Bethany introduced an 'I as rational':

> I always have it in the back of my mind what if he changed and then I really regret that my own dad wasn't there. I had a lot of those moments where what if, what if, and then I realised when I had my daughter, if he can't even do it for his own grandchild, like for me in this situation, I just can't put her [pause]. And it's just the feeling of putting someone else through it, like I can't put her through – I've been an idiot and it's been a long time. Rationally I feel ashamed even saying it. I know from a rational point of view it's just crazy but yeah, I just didn't want her to grow up with that conflict of oh grandad, but I know him, but I love him, but I thought no, it's better if she just doesn't have him. [Int: yeah] Yeah, and it was easier to make the decision for someone else than it was for myself. I've had such a lot of conflict about it
>
> *(Bethany)*

The 'I as rational' exists in dialogue with 'I as hopeful for change' and 'I as fearful of regret', ultimately concluded by naming the conflict. The voice poem shows this dialogical interplay of voices:

> *I had a lot of those moments where what if, what if*
> *I realised when I had my daughter, if he can't even do it for his own grandchild, like for me...*
> *I just can't put her...*
> *I can't put her through*
> *I've been an idiot*
> *I feel ashamed even saying it.*

I know from a rational point of view it's just crazy
I know him
I love him
I thought no
I've had such a lot of conflict about it

As I explored already in this chapter, one strategy of narrating precarity or ontological insecurity can be through a story of a battle. Here, there is a seeming battle between rationality and emotion. This continued to thread through Bethany's account:

Bethany: it's not normal, it's not rational to want contact with the person who's done that. But [pause] you know, you can't... it's really messy when it happens to you because you're confused about all the societal messages about love and family and blood and blood's thicker than water and [sigh] you know? So I just don't think people would – unless they'd had, or even maybe if they'd had a life themselves that hadn't quite gone to plan, maybe they would understand more. But I'd just be too scared that they would think I'm you know, just not – I don't... [sigh] not thinking the right things
Int: Not thinking the right things?
Bethany: Well you know, even that. Even thinking oh my god you know, my dad walked me down the aisle at my wedding. It's even hard to explain why I did that when all those things have happened but [pause] yeah it's hard to explain – even I'm not sure why

When Bethany said, 'I always have it in the back of my mind, what if he changed, and then I really regret that my own dad wasn't there', this is a voice of hope that one day her dad may change and she may regret cutting him out of her life. However, the voice of hope co-exists with a voice of shame: 'I've been an idiot and it's been a long time. Rationally I feel ashamed even saying it. I know from a rational point of view it's just crazy but yeah'. This is a story of an internal battle through which the process of articulating a voice of hope alongside a voice of rationality produced a complicated story to tell that Bethany was aware risked positioning her as 'crazy'. This could also be understood as hermeneutical injustice – a form of epistemic injustice where there is a gap in hermeneutic resources between speaker and listener, sometimes meaning that even the speaker themselves may not understand their reality fully, and that they probably have difficulty finding a way to coherently communicate it in intelligible ways to others.

Narrating survival when there is potential to be misunderstood

Bethany's awareness of the potential to be misunderstood is evident, not only by the way that she acknowledged the risk of sounding crazy, but she also pointed to that risk in other ways. For example, she said, 'in my professional life I never tell anyone'. She explained that it is 'hard to understand from the outside', and that it is 'hard to explain' because people might think that she is 'not thinking the right things'. In the absence of adequate narratives, it is important to note that women are not entirely failed. Other researchers have also found when researching issues such as recovery from rape and sexual abuse (Woodiwiss, 2014), recovery from, and/or living with depression (Chowdhury et al., 2020; Lafrance, 2007) and distress about birth experiences (Chadwick et al., 2014), women find creative, nuanced and strategic ways of communicating their stories. However, as other feminist scholars have suggested, it requires nuanced, critical and sensitive listening in order to hear women's voices, particularly voices that challenge dominant storytelling practices (Chadwick, 2009; Doucet & Mauthner, 2008). McKenzie-Mohr and Lafrance (2011) suggested that 'in the absence of adequate narratives, dominant scripts take hold so easily, swallowing up the nuances of speakers' meanings' (p. 63).

Here, Bethany was aware of the potential for her meaning to be misunderstood, so to navigate this hermeneutic gap, she took up a both/and position so that the nuances in her story had a chance of being heard. She articulated stories where she explicitly voiced multiple I positions. For example,

> he's done horrific things to me. You know he strangled me in public. It doesn't mean – it's not normal, it's not rational to want contact with the person who's done that. But [pause] you know, you can't... it's really messy when it happens to you.

She also falls to phrases like 'it's really messy' and her sentences drop off, for example, 'it doesn't mean – it's not normal' or the 'I' speaking position drops off and she uses 'you': 'it's really messy when it happens to you... you're confused'. These storytelling practices point to the challenge of articulating stories that dominant narrative frameworks do not make space for. Similarly, Nadine reflected on the pull for her father to be in her life.

> there are times, even now, when I look at people and they've got both their parents coming to see them at uni or they're being helped by their parents and I just think, would I have him back just so I could have that stability and he could do everything like now when things go wrong in the house, part of me is like oh I kind of wish he was still there, cos like nothing ever

went wrong when he was there. Like he'd just get it fixed straight away, and yeah, the reality of him not being around even though rationally I know god, I don't want him back ever. I don't want to see him ever. But it's that kind of pull, because they're still your parent as well, and that kind of, I don't know like you almost still want them to be proud of you and to love you, even though that's not gonna happen, but there's still that innate drive to just yeah

(Nadine)

Nadine, like Bethany, also negotiated a precarious storytelling context where there was a risk that her lived reality may not be understood, or, where parts of her voiced account did not align with a rational voice. Nadine said 'it's that kind of pull, because they're still your parent.... There's still that innate drive to just yeah'. While words fail Nadine and she fell to silence here, the innate pull still exists in contradiction with voice that stated 'god, I don't want him back ever'. Explicitly narrating and naming this as a 'pull' is a way of asking the listener to do the work of dwelling in, tuning in, and staying with the inconsistencies in her story. It helps to do what Chadwick defines as resisting 'efforts to "smooth over" ambiguity and discontinuities' in women's storytelling' (Chadwick, 2017, p. 71). Other feminist scholars have also called for 'listening for, and lingering in, the spaces where language fails' (McKenzie-Mohr & Lafrance, 2011, p. 65). I wanted to listen for and linger in these spaces here. Bethany and other participants regularly fell to phrases such as, 'I don't know', 'I'm not sure why' and 'it was confusing', and other ways of filling spaces such as silences, sighs and gaps in speech, for example, 'they would think I'm you know, just not – I don't... [sigh]' *(Bethany)*. These ambiguities constitute battle stories when the contradictions *become* the focus, and the story *is* the contradiction and the push and pull.

Jasmine described meeting her father with questions for him. She described the meeting as offering closure, but she also explained that her questions were still unanswered:

I wanted to erm, sort of ask why [pause] he gave up. So I think – when I was younger I was always confused as to why he did give up, although I knew that I made excuses not to see him, I always kind of wanted him to want me, and kind of stop it all and stuff, and obviously that never happened. Eventually he got sick. So I used to say 'oh I don't wanna come round because I didn't like the food' but that wouldn't mean that I wouldn't want to not see him, cos if he'd offered to take me somewhere I would have been fine, but he never did and so I just never saw him again. One of my things was 'why did you just never speak to me again?' but it – I'm still confused now, because I remember having all my nightmares and being so worried that he would come back, but then at the same time being so hurt that he rejected me in the first place. All really confusing. So that was one of my big things was why would you ever give up on someone? Especially your child?

(Jasmine)

By directly naming the confusion, her story points again to a battle between rationality and emotion. The articulation of that battle through explicitly voicing confusion, and therefore, confusion and contradiction becoming the foregrounded story, can be understood as one way of storying ontological insecurity in a way that invites and asks the listener to stay with the insecurity and ambiguities that are central to these navigations that are not only located in the past but that are also ongoing.

Sense-making when things don't make sense

This section focuses on how participants narrated uncertainties and tensions between 'I' positions, especially when stories included participants in a process of trying to make sense of things that did not seem to make sense. In this section, I consider the strategies participants employed in order to have their accounts still heard, even though they contained gaps, silences and ambiguities. I use examples of participants trying to make sense of who was responsible and accountable for the violence they experienced in order to explore this. I introduced Sonia in Chapter 6. Sonia experienced her father's violence towards her mother and occasionally his violence towards her and her sibling, as her mother would re-direct his violence towards them. In the interview, Sonia grappled with how to hold her father accountable for the violence while also feeling a sense of blame towards her mother for not protecting her.

> I do kind of blame my mum and feel more feelings of anger towards my mum, even though the violence came from my dad. I mean I know there was a couple of times, she didn't really hit us or anything it was just throwing things really but yeah I feel like she didn't protect us and I feel like she could have put more effort into their relationship to make him happier
>
> *(Sonia)*

> I kind of feel more angry now as an adult because I look and I think, if I were a mother and the same thing happened, I'd like to think – and I know it is difficult, but I'd like to think that [pause]. Because I feel like sometimes she'd keep the violence away from her, like the violence and the aggression away from her. So she'd tell my dad that we'd been naughty, or something like that, which I look and I feel that is so bad, that's the other

thing, when I read some stories, normally you read that the mother would do anything to protect the children, and I found the opposite in my case. I think I have a question as to why

(Sonia)

In Sonia's account, it is a struggle to hold her father accountable for the violence that he used. It made sense to her that her father would be responsible for the violence he used. However, she also held a truth that her mother did not protect them, meaning she felt more anger towards her mother. Nadine also spoke about these tensions in how she made sense of accountability. There were times when she would stand up for her mother in the face of violent attacks from her father, but her mother did not do the same for her.

> my dad used to like, I don't know why he did it, he used to drive and just drive with me and mum in the car. And then make me get out and then drive away. And he always came back – he always came back and got me but it was like that 10 minutes which feels like hours when you're a child. And you think this is it, I've finally been so bad that he's just gonna abandon me here. That used to make me really upset. He used to do it to my mum as well, but I – when he'd drive off and leave her, I'd be screaming and shouting and crying and begging him in the car, like don't leave her there. So – which he always did. I never could quite get my head around that as a child – he never left me there, but I just thought every time that this would be the last time [Int: mhmm]. Then I was always sad when I got back in the car because it didn't seem like my mum had put up a fight like I did

(Nadine)

The focus of these stories is a push and pull; as I explored earlier in this chapter, there is a tussle between what participants often called a 'rational' voice and a voice that was shaped by emotion. Sonia and Nadine both reflected:

> I look and I feel that is so bad, that's the other thing, when I read some stories, normally you read that the mother would do anything to protect the children

(Sonia)

> I remember being angry with my mum but never really with my dad. Like internally I'd be cross with my mum. Because I guess what he said – that she was useless and pathetic and weak, and it was just like his voice. But it was her that I'd be angry with, even though she never did anything to me. She never hurt me in any way, she just let him do that, or like I don't know

(Nadine)

In Chapter 5, I explored how gendered discourses about mothering and ideal femininity shaped the stories women told, particularly in the context of 'growing up' and navigating intimate partner relationships, mothering and family life. These narrative resources of mothering and femininity also shaped how they narrated and made sense of their relationships with their own mothers. It is assumed that the role of the mother is to protect the child. This provides a narrative resource through which young adult women can talk about their mothers and make sense of accountability or responsibility for the violence and their lack of protection as children. While this failure to protect narrative resource was re-inscribed *through* their stories, some participants also rejected this location of blame on their mothers too. I want to turn attention to how participants negotiated this re-inscription and rejection. Sonia continued to try to make sense of this tension:

> I look and I think, if I were a mother and the same thing happened, I'd like to think – and I know it is difficult, but I'd like to think that [extended pause].
>
> *(Sonia)*

Sonia acknowledged, 'I know it's difficult', and then her sentence dropped into silence and her story changed focus. The way that her sentence drops off and the way that there are disjunctions in her talk suggests that her articulation of blame is constrained. The maternal protectiveness discourse, although useful in part, may also be insufficient and may not capture the full reality of Sonia's experience. Dominant narrative frameworks about maternal protectiveness and mother–child relationships had failed her in this instance. She went on to say:

> even though it was him who was violent I just feel that she had more of a responsibility and she could have actually, I dunno, sounds not very – you know, made him happy. But she was just so selfish in so many ways
>
> *(Sonia)*

Again, the way that she reflected, 'I dunno, sounds not very – you know, made him happy', suggests that there are significant limitations to maternal protectiveness narrative resources, as Sonia fell to gaps, silences, uncertainties and hesitancies in her account. These gaps, silences and hesitancies suggest there is a precarity of narrating something that does not appear to make sense – something that is characterised by a to-and-fro, a sense that a mother was selfish and failed to protect and a knowledge that she herself was a victim too. Sonia fell to silence and checked in with me (e.g. 'It sounds not very – you know?'). This almost served as a way of recognising that it may not make sense – it is hard and maybe narratively impossible to make sense of in a coherent, integrated way.

Some existing literature has explored similar themes in relation to adults' experiences of mother–child relationships in domestic violence, suggesting that mothers and children are disadvantaged by gendered socio-structural forces that provide homogenous and sometimes harmful scripts. Moulding et al. (2015) interviewed adults about growing up with domestic violence. They found some adults reflect that their mother may not have protected them, but they were also aware of the emotional work involved in trying to make sense of this 'failure' to protect. My analysis here suggests that even though young adults can hold some anger and blame towards their mothers, they still struggle to account for why their mothers did not leave or did not do more to protect them.

For most of the women I interviewed, it was an ongoing battle to make sense of blame and accountability. Directly drawing attention to the challenge of telling a coherent story that is readable by others can be seen as a way of re-inscribing these dominant narrative resources in order to be heard while simultaneously rejecting them. Thus, I consider that actively voicing the challenge is a way of inviting the listener to 'stay with' the struggle. Nadine's account evidences this:

> I think it's just like the magnitude that you try and get your head around, it's just impossible, you can't. But then I'm still like not angry with my dad? And even I don't understand that cos I feel like I should be
>
> *(Nadine)*

It is the magnitude of the abuse Nadine experienced from her father that is impossible to make sense of. Nadine used the interview space to question herself – to question why she was not angry with her dad. This can again be understood as a form of hermeneutical injustice as even Nadine herself struggles to comprehend these contradictory I positions, never mind finding a way to intelligibly communicate it to me. This narrative challenge points to a hermeneutical injustice that happens when there is no shared sense-making resource to draw on between speaker and listener, meaning sometimes the speaker themself may struggle to understand her own experience fully (Fricker, 2007).

From a dialogical view, when we speak, we do not speak in monologue; we speak in dialogue. However, in a social and cultural context that privileges monologue and single storylines that are unchanging, women risk their dialogues being simplified, and the less-dominant voices risk being erased. The voice poem from the above extract draws attention to this dialogue.

I'm still not like angry with my dad?
I don't understand that
I should be

Nadine's account is reflective of other participants, too. It consists of 'self-negotiations, self-contradictions and self-integrations' (Hermans, 2001, p. 252) as she attempted to story a coherent story – to make sense of something that did not appear to make sense. Her question of why she was not angry with her dad, in dialogue with a sense that she 'should' be, points to the power of external voices that do not align with her experience. Her sense that she should be angry and should hold her father accountable for his violence would, in this story, mean relinquishing the anger she felt towards her mother for the part Nadine felt her mother played in not stopping the violence. Through this story, it is difficult to hold her father accountable when maternal protectiveness discourses also shape a voice that felt let down by her mother. If she tells a story of anger with her father, then she does not get to voice the sense of being unprotected and let down. The intertwined and fluid way that these I positions exist means that it is not possible to separate Nadine's co-existing voices here, and it is necessary to attend to all of what she says. On one hand, the inconsistency compromises a sense of logic in her story. However, the act of telling these stories of conflict and contradiction can be looked at as a strategy to invite the listener to hear and stay with the multiplicity.

Summary

This chapter has explored the creative narrative strategies women used in order for their more precariously told stories to be heard. I view this precarious work as important to attend to because it is precisely these unheard or more marginalised voices that often become sidelined, dismissed or pathologised in particular contexts. I understand these stories as characterised by ambiguity, hesitancy, inconsistency and sometimes fragmentation. These kinds of qualities can sometimes mean women's stories become considered untrustworthy or not credible. I understand this through a lens of epistemic injustice, particularly hermeneutical injustice, which occurs when there is a gap in hermeneutical resources between speaker and listener or between social groups. This can mean that sometimes the speaker herself cannot find a way to comprehend what she wants to say, never mind find a way of making it intelligible and communicable for others. This can mean that the speaker risks her voice becoming seen and heard as lacking credibility.

Considered in a dialogical way, there is an important meaning here. Susan Brison, in her personal account and philosophical theorisation of recovery in the aftermath of trauma and violence, suggested that 'in order to construct self-narratives we need not only the words with which to tell our stories but also an audience willing and able to hear us and to understand our words as we intend them' (Brison, 2002, p. 51). Brison powerfully recognises the relational and contextual way that we narrate the self , as well as the importance of epistemic justice. We do not tell stories in isolation, but rather, we need listeners who are willing to listen and able to understand what we are trying to say. When what we are trying to say is characterised by tension, conflict or uncertainty, this becomes a challenge. The very construction of the stories in this chapter relies on a sense of tension, a to-and-fro between I positions and the co-existence of multiple, sometimes contradictory, I positions. These stories do something by acting as a strategy to invite the listener in and to *stay* in rather than overlook, dismiss or simply not hear ambiguity, uncertainty and conflict.

I have explored how using metaphor can be a way of communicating to the listener that it is important to dwell in and pay attention to seemingly incongruous stories (McKenzie-Mohr & Lafrance, 2011; Woodcock, 2016). Specifically, this chapter has explored stories that were told as a 'battle' or a 'fight'. At the core of battle stories lies a push and pull and a story of conflict. Storying these accounts through a fight or battle metaphor, again, was a way of inviting the listener 'in' to the conflict that was central to the account. It is important to look at the socio-cultural context here, particularly from a gendered lens. Women speak and live in a socio-cultural context that privileges masculine and rational storylines, and, as Sara Ahmed has noted, there exists a hierarchy of emotion and logic that does not always make space for stories that are led by or which centre emotion (Ahmed, 2014). Women both re-inscribed and resisted these socio-cultural resources, which devalue emotion and privilege logic. To negotiate this and, in some senses, attempt to mitigate the potential for devaluing the emotion, participants explicitly spoke from both emotion and logic voices, and explicitly named the conflict when they did. Speaking from a rational voice can provide women with a credible story that is fixed and a story through which others can understand them. However, participants often explicitly expressed the risk that others would not understand, sometimes even questioning themselves, suggesting a kind of ontological insecurity whereby their own sense of self and subjective reality is not reflected in the relational and social environments around them. This can further embed a logic–emotion binary, meaning that uncertainties and hesitancies are more challenging to narrate.

Women used creative strategies to articulate multiple I positions by using metaphors, occupying both/and positions, and taking time to check in that I understood, pausing to invite me to 'dwell in' the ambiguities they expressed, or simply dropping to silence. The strategies I have explored in this chapter were used despite and because of the limited available narrative resources for the women I interviewed. I also consider that the emotion–logic binary that this chapter examines produces and contributes to epistemic injustices where women are disadvantaged, particularly if the stories they tell contain voices that contradict logic. Participants were aware of the risk that their stories might be misinterpreted or misunderstood, and I have explored how some of these creative strategies functioned to directly acknowledge multiple

I positions, in an effort to invite the listener to 'dwell in' the tensions. Tuning into tensions and contradictions can make for uncomfortable listening, but to really tune in and stay there demands a commitment to dwelling in these tensions, and noticing when there is an invitation to do so.

References

Adkins, L. (2001). Cultural feminization: "Money, sex and power" for women. *Signs*, 26(3), 669–695. https://doi.org/10.2307/3175536

Ahmed, S. (2014). *The cultural politics of emotion* (2nd ed.). Edinburgh University Press.

Alcoff, L. (2018). *Rape and resistance*. Polity Press.

Baerger, D. R., & McAdams, D. P. (1999). Life story coherence and its relation to psychological well-being. *Narrative Inquiry*, 9(1), 69–96. https://doi.org/10.1075/NI.9.1.05BAE/CITE/REFWORKS

Baker, J. (2010). Great expectations and post-feminist accountability: Young women living up to the "successful girls" discourse. *Gender and Education*, 22(1), 1–15. https://doi.org/10.1080/09540250802612696

Beck, U., & Beck-Gernsheim, E. (2002). *Individualization: Institutionalized individualism and its social and political consequences*. SAGE Publications.

Bondi, L. (2014). Feeling insecure: A personal account in a psychoanalytic voice. *Social & Cultural Geography*, 15(3), 332–350. https://doi.org/10.1080/14649365.2013.864783

Brison, S. (2002). *Aftermath: Violence and the remaking of a self*. Princeton University Press.

Cambridge Dictionary, Precarious English Meaning. (2024). Cambridge Dictionary. https://dictionary.cambridge.org/dictionary/english/precarious

Chadwick, R. (2017). Embodied methodologies: Challenges, reflections and strategies. *Qualitative Research*, 17(1), 54–74. https://doi.org/10.1177/1468794116656035

Chadwick, R. J. (2009). Between bodies, cultural scripts and power: The reproduction of birthing subjectivities in home-birth narratives. *Subjectivity*, 27(1), 109–133. https://doi.org/10.1057/sub.2009.1

Chadwick, R. J., Cooper, D., & Harries, J. (2014). Narratives of distress about birth in South African public maternity settings: A qualitative study. *Midwifery*, 30(7), 862–868. https://doi.org/10.1016/J.MIDW.2013.12.014

Chowdhury, N., Gibson, K., & Wetherell, M. (2020). Polyphonies of depression: The relationship between voices-of-the-self in young professional women aka "top girls." *Health*, 24(5), 773–790. https://doi.org/10.1177/1363459319846934

Doucet, A., & Mauthner, N. S. (2008). What can be known and how? Narrated subjects and the listening guide. *Qualitative Research*, 8(3), 399–409. https://doi.org/10.1177/1468794106093636

Fricker, M. (2007). *Epistemic injustice: Power and the ethics of knowing*. Oxford University Press.

Giddens, A. (1991). *Modernity and self-identity. Self and society in the late modern age*. Polity Press.

Gill, R., & Orgad, S. (2018). The amazing bounce-backable woman: Resilience and the psychological turn in neoliberalism. *Sociological Research Online*, 23(2), 477–495. https://doi.org/10.1177/1360780418769673

Gill, R., & Scharff, C. (2011). *New femininities: Postfeminism, neoliberalism, and subjectivity*. Palgrave Macmillan.

Herman, J. (2015). *Trauma and recovery: The aftermath of violence - from domestic abuse to political terror*. Basic Books.

Hermans, H. J. M. (2001). The dialogical self: Toward a theory of personal and cultural positioning. *Culture & Psychology*, 7(3), 243–281. https://doi.org/10.1177/1354067X0173001

Hydén, M. (2014). The teller-focused interview: Interviewing as a relational practice. *Qualitative Social Work: Research and Practice*, 13(6), 795–812. https://doi.org/10.1177/1473325013506247

Lafrance, M. N. (2007). A bitter pill: A discursive analysis of women's medicalized accounts of depression. *Journal of Health Psychology*, 12(1), 127–140. https://doi.org/10.1177/1359105307071746

Laing, R. D. (2010). *The divided self*. Penguin.

McKenzie-Mohr, S., & Lafrance, M. N. (2011). Telling stories without the words: 'Tightrope talk' in women's accounts of coming to live well after rape or depression. *Feminism & Psychology*, 21(1), 49–73. https://doi.org/10.1177/0959353510371367

McRobbie, A. (2004). Post-feminism and popular culture. *Feminist Media Studies*, 4(3), 255–264. https://doi.org/10.1080/1468077042000309937

McRobbie, A. (2015). Notes on the perfect: Competitive femininity in neoliberal times. *Australian Feminist Studies*, 30(83), 3–20. https://doi.org/10.1080/08164649.2015.1011485

Moulding, N. T., Buchanan, F., & Wendt, S. (2015). Untangling self-blame and mother-blame in women's and children's perspectives on maternal protectiveness in domestic violence: Implications for practice. *Child Abuse Review*, 24(4), 249–260. https://doi.org/10.1002/car.2389

Rose, N. (1992). "Governing the enterprising self." In P. Heelas & P. Morris (Eds.), *The values of the enterprise culture: The moral debate* (pp. 141–164). Routledge.

Rose, N. (2010). 'Screen and intervene': Governing risky brains. *History of the Human Sciences*, 23(1), 79–105. https://doi.org/10.1177/0952695109352415

Woodcock, C. (2016). The listening guide. *International Journal of Qualitative Methods*, 15(1), 1–10. https://doi.org/10.1177/1609406916677594

Woodiwiss, J. (2014). Beyond a single story: The importance of separating 'harm' from 'wrongfulness' and 'sexual innocence' from 'childhood' in contemporary narratives of childhood sexual abuse. *Sexualities*, 17(1–2), 139–158. https://doi.org/10.1177/1363460713511104

8
TOWARD EPISTEMIC JUSTICE
Embodied and reflexive listening

Introduction

Listening to people's stories is not a neutral or detached and distanced process. Anyone who works with people's life stories engages with the material in embodied, emotional and personal ways. In the previous chapter, I explored the narrative work participants did and the creative strategies they employed to invite me, the listener, 'into' their stories and hear parts of their stories that were perhaps more difficult to articulate. In this chapter, I consider that the practice and process of listening continues beyond the interview itself. I draw on concepts of embodiment and reflexivity to reflect on my experience working with voice poems. I understand embodiment as a way of being. A way of inhabiting the multiple aspects of our lived experience through the body. It is an understanding that mind and body are connected and inseparable. In previous chapters, I explored epistemic injustice, drawing on Miranda Fricker's conceptualisations of hermeneutical and testimonial injustice. I have examined how both these concepts can be applied to the women I interviewed as I understood their accounts. In this chapter, I explore how the methods I used, and myself as the researcher, were key parts of addressing and drawing attention to these epistemic injustices.

I have come to consider voice poems, in part, as a 'way in' to our own stories and selves, and I have come to consider this as a fundamental part of knowledge generation. This chapter is about my own experience listening, what I learnt from reflecting on my listening practices, and how I was changed by listening. I think about *how* I listened and consider my own role in the knowledge-generation process. I hope that this chapter speaks to readers who are, like myself, researchers, psychotherapists or counsellors – or

DOI: 10.4324/9781003393160-8

indeed, anybody whose life requires them to listen attentively and sensitively to the life stories of others. In this chapter, I delve more into my personal experiences of working with the data, and I hope this provides some insights into what the analysis process was like and that it was not a neat or linear process. I intentionally want to show some of the messiness and stickiness of working with stories that can be difficult to hear. Stories that can remind one of one's own history, and data that somehow draws you in over and over again. This is not a self-interested chapter, but rather, I hope to show how attending to these personal processes in reflexive, mindful and curious ways can support knowledge generation, be generative for understanding parts of the self and be valuable in terms of working toward epistemic justice when listening to women's accounts of trauma and violence.

Bodymind listening as work toward epistemic justice

In 2016, when I started envisioning this research project and started my PhD, I did not have much experience using artful forms of inquiry, and I did not set out to use poems as part of my analysis. However, as I engaged with literature surrounding the value and need for a dialogical and relational approach to listening (for example, Chadwick, 2017; Doucet & Mauthner, 2008; Phoenix & Pattynama, 2006), I discovered the Listening Guide. In some respects, this was the first 'hook'. The production of poems through the Listening Guide appealed to me as it spoke to my artistic and creative self (notably less nurtured since I was a teen and a part of me I am trying to connect more with as an adult) and my academic self (significantly more foregrounded through adulthood so far). However, I also realised that our creative, artful selves and our academic selves are not binary identities. The voice poems I produced as part of the analysis, and that I have shared in Chapters 5–7, acted as both a source of knowledge and a form of artful inquiry. I became aware that the poems I created were the stories of participants, and at the same time, I was re-storying accounts that were entangled with my own stories. Consequently, the analysis process was also a process of re-examining parts of myself. It was also a process of asking questions about what made some voices more able to be heard and what kinds of circumstances contributed to the erasure, marginalisation or silencing of others. These were, and are, questions I still explore in relation to myself as well as the accounts of participants.

The body – *my* body – became a crucial source of knowledge as I grappled with these questions around epistemic justice. I think of bodymind listening through working with voice poems as a unique opportunity to examine questions of power and knowledge, to see and feel in a different way, how particular voices get foregrounded and others do not and to ask what epistemic justice may look like or feel like, as a listener. Other qualitative and feminist researchers have also argued that research is an embodied practice and process (Chadwick, 2017; Ellingson, 2016; Fox, 2015). In other words, they have put forward the perspective that how we make sense of and theorise the stories we work with can extend beyond words. The more that I worked with the data in this research and the more I reflected on my own personal life and process at the time, I realised that the two were very interrelated, almost inseparably so. Reflexivity became not a one-off journal writing session or identification of how my own positionality informed the interviewer–interviewee relationship, although I did do both of these things. Rather than a mind-based activity that relies on declaring and engaging with a unitary self, I came to understand researchers – and myself – as dialogical selves that are both *affected by,* and that *affect,* the material we work with.

In this chapter, I draw on Lenz Taguchi's (2012) theorisations of the bodymind of the researcher to explore how my affective and emotional responses to this research project were important sources of knowledge. In doing so, I consider thinking as not a 'mind' activity, but it is a transcorporeal act in which bodies are not passive tools, but bodies are always affecting and being affected by each other. In Chapter 3, in introducing Dialogical Self Theory, I briefly introduced the idea of Cartesian logic – the idea that the mind is separate from the body. This Cartesian logic is underpinned by the idea that the mind should somehow be in control of the body (Launeanu & Kwee, 2018). This dualistic mind–body logic also promotes a disengagement with the body by privileging mind-based thought and logic and de-privileging body-based knowledge and wisdom. In Chapter 3, I explained I aim to embrace a non-Cartesian approach in this work. Embodiment can, therefore, be viewed as a way of embracing a non-Cartesian approach to mind and body.

This chapter offers some examples of how I worked with and was changed by the stories I listened to. I use some examples of the voice poems and transcript extracts I shared in the previous three chapters to explore how my own embodied involvement with the research process became an important source of knowledge and enabled me to examine discomfort as a 'hook'. I consider voice poems as a 'hook' – a 'way in' to our affective, embodied and emotional selves. Here, I draw on Singleton's (2020) conceptualisation of 'hooks' as the things that draw us in and the things that we might get 'stuck on' (p. 5), and that these 'hooks' are opportunities to examine the self. Aspects of voice poems that acted as 'hooks' included where the hooks were clearly (and sometimes not clear at the time) visible and viscerally felt in ways that I did not connect with when I engaged with the full non-fragmented interview transcripts. These 'hooks' offered reflexive opportunities, which threaded through my analysis, and offered opportunities to re-examine myself, enabling me to 'dwell in' these poems and examine these places of discomfort in bolder ways than I suspect I would have done if I was working with interview transcripts as standalone texts.

Listeners as dialogical and always-changing selves

Central to this book, and how I have made sense of the data from my interviews with women, is Dialogical Self Theory (Hermans, 2001, 2022). As I hope has been evident, this theory assumes that being human is about being in relation, and it is through human relationships and dialogue that we come into existence (Graf-Taylor, 2012). As such, to be human is to be always in flux, always changing and always coming into existence in our particular social, cultural and relational contexts. A dialogical philosophy is an assumption that the boundaries of the self are diffused with those of the 'other' – we are always at meeting points in relation with others, always impacted and affected; therefore, the 'other' is not an object, they are a subject, coming into existence through dialogue and relationship.

I found that working with voice poems presented a unique opportunity to reflect on how we as researchers might come to understand more about our multiple selves and more about ourselves as dialogical beings. I became interested in how the voice poems and my analysis of them was shaped by and entangled with my own material. I should say that I, among other feminist qualitative researchers, do not see this as a problem to rectify or fix by somehow finding a way of removing myself or bracketing myself from the data with the assumption that objectivity exists and is the desired outcome (Del Busso, 2007; Finlay, 2002; Lazard & McAvoy, 2020; Wilkinson, 1988). Rather, I explore the idea that engaging with material in this creative, reflexive and embodied way enables a resistance against theorising the self as a unitary subject. It has the potential to make available the possibility of considering the self as dialogical, multiple and coming into being through relation and dialogue with others. My learning from this research project is that this can be the case for both the material we work with and for our own selves as researchers. This is an epistemological commitment that is especially important in domestic violence research, where women's survivor/victim accounts may often be smoothened out (Alcoff, 2018) and where researcher reflexivity risks becoming a mind-based activity that assumes a unitary 'self' instead of a self that is constituted by an orchestration of multiple voices and selves (Lenz Taguchi, 2012).

In the next two sections of this chapter, I offer two examples that illustrate these reflections and learnings. I draw on examples from two voice poems from the interviews with Bethany and Frances. These voice poems held resonance for me and challenged my own understanding of myself while acting as opportunities to further understand the data I was working with. Through sharing my workings with these poems, I draw on a bodymind transcorporeal conceptualisation of self (Lenz Taguchi, 2012) to show how parts of myself came into being in new and different ways through this process of re-storying of stories through poems. I explore how this became an important part of the analytical process. I want to be clear that by offering interpretations of these voice poems, as I have done throughout the previous three chapters, I do not claim access to one particular 'truth' or an 'authentic voice' of either myself or the participants. Rather, I lean towards a lens of multiplicity, in keeping with Dialogical Self Theory. I present stories in a way that shows they were co-constructed and can always be open to reinterpretations and new understandings.

Listening as a slow process: encountering discomfort and what we might learn if we slow down

One of the voice poems that perhaps was most impactful and resonated most with me long after creating the poem is from my interview with Bethany. I was particularly struck by how seeing the visual voice poem and working with it produced a visceral response in me, and I found myself returning to it many times, sometimes unable to leave it to one side. It is from a part of the interview where Bethany is talking about how she had continued to try to maintain contact with her father long after her parents had separated and how she continued to be let down by him when he did not show up. Bethany spoke about her capacity to rationalise that her father is 'bad' and at the same time, her desire to maintain contact with him for fear of losing him. In Chapter 7, I explored there being a kind of hermeneutical injustice where parts of Bethany's knowledge and reality were seemingly difficult to communicate in an intelligible way to me as the listener or to 'anyone'. I saw there was a gap between hermeneutic resources, which produced an epistemic injustice that was shaped by a lack of shared tools of social interpretation. It was, in some ways, incomprehensible that she should want to keep her father in her life after all the violence she endured from him. At the same time, she *did* want to keep her father in her life. This is part of the voice poem I constructed from the interview with Bethany, which continued to stay with me long after I created it:

> *you can totally rationalise this person is bad.*
> *You're brought up thinking that's my dad –*
> *if I don't –*
> *if I don't,*
> *if I lose contact with him*
> *I lose, that's my dad.*
> *You let me down again and that's enough*
> *I never want to see you ever again.*

To me, this poem showed the dialogical relationship between a voice of rationality ('this person is bad'), a voice that consists of emotional entanglements of hope and fear ('I lose… that's my dad') and a voice that expressed 'rational' resistance and pushes back against emotion ('you let me down and that's enough'). The process of creating the poem itself was creative and embodied. I did it 'by hand', meaning that I printed all the transcripts out, took up a lot of space on the floor in my home with pages of transcripts and coloured pens, noting where I felt resonances and where I saw narrative resources shaping different I positions. This creative and embodied process allowed me to work with the data in a physically and emotionally close way. I found that creating breaks in speech and distinguishing between I positions in a visual and tangible way allowed space for me to see a visible representation of these breaks and shifts in the direction of 'I'. These spaces in text also invited me in – me, my body and my emotions. I found myself reading lines several times, sometimes I reflected on my own history and sometimes I dreamt about my own memories, uncovering parts of myself in new and different ways. I wondered why I, too, had struggled with navigating similar feelings. When I thought about discussing this poem in supervision or with my peers, I found myself wanting to show it to others, but having no words to describe what it meant. My body filled the silences here as I noticed I could not easily put the research down.

Although I did not necessarily notice it at the time, I became stuck. My body was tired from trying to move quickly past the stuckness, as if glazing over it and ignoring the discomfort meant that it did not exist. In part, this was a familiar pattern for me – leaning into being busy and 'doing', particularly when there is something difficult happening that feels hard to attend to. However, this was something to do with the data and something related to this particular voice poem. I became stuck in this story and stuck between the lines of the poem. This stuckness had a quality of discomfort that prevented me from 'doing' anything with my meaning-making and with the poem. I sometimes put the work down completely and stepped away. At the same time, I tried to push myself as quickly as possible to the end of the project so that I did not have to 'stay with' this discomfort and whatever I may uncover if I stayed long enough to find out. I had a supervisor who, gently and with care, would often stop me mid-rush and ask, 'Why are you rushing? What is this about?'. My strategies for pushing past discomfort included hiking to the summit of mountains, walking as far as I could, wearing my shoes down and pushing my body to the point of injury or pain or trying to shrink my body so it wouldn't have to feel. So I had no energy left until I had to pause. Until my body did not give me much choice. These were very embodied cues to pause and slow down. My efforts to push through resulted in a knee injury that eventually meant I stopped running. Stopping nourishing my body sufficiently so that I did not feel emotions so intensely meant that I eventually did not have the energy to hike, so again, my body gave me little choice but to slow down. These 'pause' days eventually became gentler days, where I did my best to 'stay with' what had been stirred in me. These were days where I attempted to examine by 'staying with' (Haraway, 2016) rather than pushing past.

The question my supervisor would sometimes ask, 'Why are you rushing? What is this about?' is one that I returned to often, in hindsight. It has become a central question that supports my own self-understanding, and that also supports my sense-making of Bethany's account. Bethany's story contained aspects that were close to my own story. Working with this material, and particularly this aspect of the interview, sometimes prompted memories or reflections that I had not remembered or considered before. This poem felt powerful and weighty, and raw and fragile, all at once, and it stayed with me even when I paused, perhaps especially when I paused. These times of pausing gave space to tune more into the dialogical interplay between the voices of rationality and emotion. Through doing this, I noticed that I also developed a greater capacity to 'be with' myself. I was better able to find words to write about how I made sense of Bethany's account, and the stuckness shifted. In some ways, you might see that I found a hermeneutical resource in this voice poem, which provided a way of making my own experience more intelligible and more comprehensible to myself.

Drawing on Wilson's (2018) conceptualisation of stories in our research that 'haunt' us, this poem drew me in, in haunting ways. This haunting affect refers to stories that invite the reader/listener 'in' in ways that stay with us (Wilson, 2018). As Wilson (2018) notes, the production and form of poems acted as a creative and alternative form of storying findings that did not look like the 'conventional academic publication or output' (p. 1214), meaning that stories stay with and 'haunt' the reader/audience, 'provoking empathy and potentially action' (p. 1214). However, this haunting impact was not a process by which the poems did something *to* me; rather, the process was dialogical and relational. The way in which I was *affected by* the story, and how *I affected* the re-storying of the story, was a product of my existence in *relationship* with the research process (LaMarre, 2021), and a product of bodymind transcorporeality (Lenz Taguchi, 2012).

Staying with stuckness

In this section of the chapter, I explore how I was affected by, and how I affected, the interpretation of my interview with Frances. In Chapter 6, I discussed how Frances narrated her recovery story centring a sense of pride and resilience that she had succeeded academically and chosen the 'better life' despite the violence she had endured from her parents and the multiple times she had not been believed when she disclosed and tried to seek help. I saw this as a form of testimonial injustice whereby her position as a child and as a girl meant that her account was less likely to be seen and heard as credible, and she was more likely to be disbelieved. This history of epistemic injustice shaped a voice of anger that, in some ways, was storied as raw and as '*too* much'. The raw and overspilling nature of the voice of anger existed in dialogue with a voice that wanted to 'do good' with her story, which, in some ways, offered a 'good' and credible recovery story to tell.

Frances was the first person that I interviewed for this project. My impressions were that I experienced Frances as articulate; she spoke about the depths of her experiences and emotions in a way that I experienced as logical and 'put together'. As far as I felt, it was not a 'messy' interview – it ran smoothly – and it almost seemed as if this was a story Frances had told many times, even though she reflected several times that she had never spoken about her childhood in this way before. In hindsight, reflecting on how I experienced this, it was almost as if Frances did extra work to ensure her account was intelligible and communicable so that I might hear. Understood in the context of a history of epistemic injustice, this makes some sense.

The set-up of our interview was interesting in this context, too. Even though I was the researcher and felt like it was my responsibility to ensure we had a good space to meet and talk, Frances did the organising. My experience was that she went above and beyond to accommodate me and ensure that my visit to her was easy and effortless. We decided to meet at her university as she was a student at the time, and this felt to us both like the most appropriate meeting space. She sent me instructions for where to park and where we would meet. Frances booked us a comfortable room at a university to do the interview in; we grabbed a coffee beforehand and had time to talk on our walk from the car park to the university room she had booked for us. The interview was contained within the time we had set aside; her story was told from beginning to end, and then she walked me back to my car afterwards. I felt like she had hosted me with care, and I was aware that usually, it would be me doing this for participants, not the other way around. I noticed I felt that I did not want to misuse her time; I wanted to listen to her story carefully, and I also noticed that I worried I would not be able to use her story to help others as she hoped.

Frances spoke about the multiple times during her childhood that she had been let down by social services and professionals who had not believed her when she told them about the abuse she was experiencing. During the interview, she spoke about her pride in her resilience, which had enabled her to survive and keep going. I had a couple of hours car journey back home, during which I felt confused about how her story was so neatly told when so much of it was a story of pain and distress. It seemed she told me her story from beginning to end in a linear way, and the ending was one of strength and resilience. On my drive home, I felt a growing sense of discomfort and confusion in the pit of my stomach, which became unsettling as I began to question whether I had listened effectively and whether I had done a good enough job at hearing her story, which contained painful and distressing experiences of loss, grief, abuse, struggle and being unheard and not believed.

This discomfort and confusion acted as a 'hook', and it persisted as I transcribed and constructed the voice poem. It became clear that there were elements of Frances' account that I had not tuned into during the interview. Frances told a story of pride and resilience, which I felt I had heard and understood during the interview. However, I became attuned to what I saw as a voice of anger through producing the voice poem. This voice of anger was related to experiences of being let down and not believed. She explained her wish to go back to services and provide feedback, in the hopes this would help others. I included some of this voice poem in Chapter 6, but I want to include more of it here to give some context for how I worked with it:

I would never want anyone to experience what I went through
I'd never want anyone to go through that
… the way I could do it is by going back to the services and giving them some feedback
I just think, well what's the point?
They let me down before
they're not gonna take my feedback seriously
I don't want to cooperate with them
I'm angry with them
I want to be able to help others
I tend to live my life without thinking about the past
… it's not something I think about
… it's not something I talk about
… it's not something that really crosses my mind.

As I created the voice poem and tried to understand the differently voiced 'I' positions, I could tune more into the anger, and my understanding was that this anger did not always align with a stable and credible account of resilience or the 'neat' way I experienced the telling of the story. I became aware that attending to my own discomfort meant attending to the rise of anger and injustice I felt in response to the multiple ways that adults in her life had indeed let down Frances. My discomfort was partly a fear that I would, too, let her down by not doing something useful with her story.

Frances' 'neat' articulation of her story became a sticking point and source of discomfort and unease, as my excessive questioning of my own listening skills did not soften. In time, through working with the shifting and fluctuating 'I' positions in the voice poem, I began to explore what I understood as the internalisation of 'external voices' (Hermans, 2001), and I examined how the socio-political context, including a history of testimonial injustice, functioned to shape the telling of the account. My own sense of injustice and discomfort, as well as my relentless questioning of my own interviewing skills, meant I was curious about Frances' 'neat' articulation of her story and why it seemed to bring about such discomfort in me that it was articulated in this way.

The way I have re-storied Frances' story through the poem shows the interplay between a voice of anger ('I don't want to cooperate with them... I'm angry with them') and a 'credible' story of recovery ('I want to be able to help others'). Frances suggested that one day, she would like to make sure that others do not experience the same as she did. Using her experience for good to help others is framed as central to a recovery story. However, a story of resilience and recovery – using her experience for good – is at odds with the anger that is also voiced, which destabilises this story of recovery. Anger is, therefore, a voice that becomes less speakable, existing on the margins or becoming silenced. It was perhaps unsurprising that I found myself somewhat stuck in how I navigated this discomfort and my own sense of anger, too. This silencing and the challenge of expressing anger in a way that does not discredit culturally valuable stories of survival or recovery pointed to the patriarchal structures that are set up to discredit the credibility of women's accounts of trauma or abuse (Brown & Burman, 1997; Fricker, 2007; Schuman & Galvez, 1996), where if women do not conform to a particular way of telling their stories (i.e. single, stable storylines, told through a unitary single voice), they may not be believed. Or even, as Frances had experienced, her gender and age meant her voice was less likely to be heard as credible. The impacts of this had been huge and long lasting for Frances.

I found that exploring this voice poem with an understanding of the gender and age-based testimonial injustice that Frances had experienced made me remember aspects of my own childhood that I rarely connected with. I found myself remembering adults in my own childhood who could have had opportunities to see that something was wrong, but they failed to name it. I found that images and memories came to the surface for me, bringing about their own layers of discomfort in ways that resonated with that pit of stomach discomfort I felt about Frances' interview. As I began to understand more of Frances' account by listening to her words, I simultaneously began to understand more of my own experiences of feeling unseen and unheard, too. In some ways, tuning into the voice of anger enabled me to connect with my own anger, too. I got curious about why I would continue to attempt to grapple with both a desire to be seen in my wholeness and a desire to make myself as small and unseen as possible, a simultaneous desire to take up space and take up no space at all.

My learning here is that tuning into my own emotional and embodied responses during the interview and when working with the voice poem provided some valuable and generative insights about both my own self as a 'becoming' human being and about the data itself. Feminist qualitative researchers who are also interested in the body and reflexivity have discussed how we might often turn away from our own emotional or embodied responses to our research material, particularly if it evokes discomfort or if it touches material of our own that we might not have attended to in such a way before (LaMarre, 2021; Singleton, 2020). Drawing on Lenz Taguchi's (2012) conceptualisation of reflexivity as a transcorporeal bodymind process, I was both *affected by* Frances' account, and I also *affected* how I re-storied her account through poems. Attending to my own discomfort enabled a route 'in' to examining the interview context and the socio-political context of Frances' history and how that shaped the voices that she spoke from. Tuning into my own responses and my own sense of unease and stuckness enabled me to examine the neatness I had heard in Frances' account. Examining my growing sense of confusion, anger and injustice enabled an interest in and resistance against a unitary conceptualisation of both myself and of Frances' account of violence.

Relational and embodied forms of knowledge

As a feminist researcher with lived experience of the issue I was researching, it might make sense that I would find myself experiencing empathy in relation to participants' accounts. This might mean that I would be more likely to 'feel' with participants. This might have been particularly available to me if elements of participants' accounts resonated with my own story. However, as I have explored in this chapter so far, I came to wonder whether 'feeling' was about more than empathy and 'feeling' could act as important and generative anchors and 'hooks'. I draw on Rachelle Chadwick's reckonings with the role of empathy and affect in feminist research. She has argued that it is important to 'move beyond the idealisation of empathy as the central affective principle in feminist research' (Chadwick, 2021, p. 1) and to stay with and attend to the 'messy ambivalences, sticky discomforts, falterings, disconnections, epistemic uncertainty and the intense feelings often evoked in/through research interactions' (Chadwick, 2021, p. 4). Through working with the voice poems I created, including the examples from the interviews with Bethany and Frances, I found that my engagement with the voice poems offered a way of working with the contrapuntal and fluctuating voices within talk that was not available through listening to the audio files or reading the transcripts as standalone texts.

The way I engaged creatively and tangibly with the material to create the poems and then make sense of them meant that I could re-examine my own experiences, coming to terms with my own contradictory voices and slowing down long enough to acknowledge them. This capacity to pause and 'be with' myself and the data shaped how I engaged with and re-storied participants' accounts through the poems. In this way, this creative process enabled me to 'become with', as I began to understand some of my own story, as well as become more curious about what this interplay of voices meant in the context of my analysis.

Turning to the body and thinking of embodied knowledge as valid, credible and trustworthy is not new (McBride, 2021). However, particularly in the sciences, including social science, there still exists a knowledge hierarchy that has historically, in Western Eurocentric contexts, devalued embodied knowledge in favour of objective 'scientific' evidence (Bondi & Fewell, 2017; Drummond, 2020; Haraway, 1988). Staying with and attending to our own 'hooks' and points of discomfort becomes an important epistemological practice, and voice poems may be one way of exploring a different way of knowing by attending to these kinds of embodied and emotional selves that come into being through working with our data. Creating poems as a reflexive analytical process enabled a way of being with data that drew me in in different ways, much more so than 'being with' and 'listening to' the interview recordings and transcripts. Engaging with the material in a visual way created opportunities to 'feel' my way in and through the stories and, at the same time, re-examine myself and my own history. As LaMarre (2021) has written, artful expressions can be a form of knowledge in feminist research, and art can be a way of 'inviting us to step into relation with that which we are exploring' (p. 2). While there can be a focus on empathy or being called to action as a social justice element of artistic inquiry (Wilson, 2018), I found that there was a humanness, an embodied-ness and a discomfort to this kind of relating that extends beyond being moved to empathise or being called to action. It is true I felt empathy, and as time has passed, I sometimes feel a call to 'do' something in response to the epistemic injustices that thread through participants' accounts. But my overriding sense is that for some of the analytical process, I was not called to *do* anything. In fact, when I did feel pulled to *do*, these were moments when it was often necessary to *be with* the material.

Working with voice poems became not only a method and a 'tool', but the poems also became an opportunity to consider the interconnectedness of methodology and epistemology. Working with voice poems offered unique opportunities to attend to and resist epistemological injustices by rejecting positivist and empiricist conceptualisations of 'authentic voice' and 'stable self'. As noted by Fox (2015), the relationship between methodology and epistemology is particularly important when working with epistemological injustices that are enabled and enacted through methodologies that erase or obscure marginalised voices. Given that I was working with voices that are typically marginalised and positioned as unstable and thus, not credible, attending to and resisting epistemological injustices was important.

Drawing on the example of working with Frances' account, voice poems can be considered a method of resistance because of the way that they enable attention to how personal stories are intertwined and situated in social, cultural and political contexts. Staying with my own discomfort as I created and made sense of the voice poem helped to dismantle the idea that we speak from one single stable voice, and this practice supported the examination of both anger and strength and survivorship in Frances' account, as well as the historical experiences of testimonial injustice. This commitment to a dialogical and relational philosophy required rejection of the concept of the rational or independent 'self'. Drawing on Haraway's (1988) feminist politics of knowledge production, my workings with the voice poems highlighted the need to keep close the assumption that knowledge is produced situationally and contextually. This resistance 'holds at its core the idea of a relational ontology in which conceptions of the separate, self-sufficient, independent, rational "self" or "individual" are rejected in favour of notions of "selves-in-relation" or "relational beings"' (Mauthner & Doucet, 2003, p. 421). This way of inviting us to pay attention, through the form of poetic inquiry and 'being with' data and ourselves, can be viewed as a resistance to epistemic injustices, by extending beyond poems as simply a 'tool' or a listening 'technique'.

Summary

As researchers, often, the 'self' is assumed to be separate and detached from our research material, and we might be encouraged to find ways of removing or bracketing ourselves so that we do not overly influence our sense-making or become biased in our conclusions. I hope this chapter has done something to explore how researchers and story-listeners can become entangled, affective, affected and intimately involved in the analysis and knowledge production processes. This chapter has explored how this is not something to avoid. Rather, it could be a process to examine and try to understand. Rather than constructing this self-involvement and relating as problematic, or as something that needs to be 'contained' or 'managed', I consider it a necessary part of theorising and connecting with the human messiness of how we are affected by that which we encounter in our research processes (Chadwick, 2021; LaMarre, 2021), and simultaneously, how we affect the material that we work with and the knowledge we produce (Lenz Taguchi, 2012).

Working with voice poems was generative and moving. It has inspired me to want to work with poems more and to attend to multivocality as a serious epistemic commitment to reduce epistemic injustice, work against epistemic violence and work towards a more epistemically just way of listening to women's accounts of trauma. Importantly for this project, the voice poems helped me to tune into the multivocality of stories, including voices that were my own, voices that were participants' and storylines that came into being through the dialogic interplay of both my own and participants' stories. This chapter has explored how a dialogical lens and bodymind reflexivity enabled me to begin to examine my own contradictory and fluctuating 'I positions', learn more about myself and re-examine parts of myself, in relation to the material I was working with. I also showed how this process enabled me to attune more and attend to the multivocality of participants' accounts as I re-storied their accounts and made sense of them through poems.

In the following final chapter, I expand on the implications of this book more broadly and offer some concluding comments. However, speaking directly to working reflexively and creatively with stories, this chapter specifically addresses how methods and listening practices have implications for domestic violence research, where survivor–victim voices tend to be smoothened out, resulting in dominant, binary narratives that risk reproducing epistemic injustices. This chapter has explored the opportunities that creative and poetic inquiry can offer, as I consider working with voice poems to be a method of resistance to epistemological injustices. I hope this chapter has offered insights into how I worked reflexively with the poems in the analytical process. Importantly, I hope it has shown how I tuned into my body using bodymind reflexivity. Reflecting on the analytical process, I consider voice poems and creative inquiry as offering unique opportunities for attending to multivocality, marginalised voices and working toward epistemic justice.

References

Alcoff, L. (2018). *Rape and resistance*. Polity Press.
Bondi, L., & Fewell, J. (2017). Getting personal: A feminist argument for research aligned to therapeutic practice. *Counselling and Psychotherapy Research*, 17(2), 113–122. https://doi.org/10.1002/capr.12102
Brown, L. S., & Burman, E. (1997). Feminist responses to the 'false memory' debate. *Feminism & Psychology*, 7(1), 7–16. https://doi.org/10.1177/0959353597071002
Chadwick, R. (2017). Embodied methodologies: Challenges, reflections and strategies. *Qualitative Research*, 17(1), 54–74. https://doi.org/10.1177/1468794116656035
Chadwick, R. (2021). On the politics of discomfort. *Feminist Theory*, 22(4), 556–574. https://doi.org/10.1177/1464700120987379
Del Busso, L. (2007). III. Embodying feminist politics in the research interview: Material bodies and reflexivity. *Feminism and Psychology*, 17(3), 309–315. https://doi.org/10.1177/0959353507079084
Doucet, A., & Mauthner, N. S. (2008). What can be known and how? Narrated subjects and the listening guide. *Qualitative Research*, 8(3), 399–409. https://doi.org/10.1177/1468794106093636
Drummond, A. (2020). Embodied Indigenous knowledges protecting and privileging indigenous peoples' ways of knowing, being and doing in undergraduate nursing education. *The Australian Journal of Indigenous Education*, 49(2), 127–134. https://doi.org/10.1017/JIE.2020.16
Ellingson, L. L. (2016). Embodied knowledge: Writing researchers' bodies into qualitative health research. *Qualitative Health Research*, 16(2), 298–310. https://doi.org/10.1177/1049732305281944
Finlay, L. (2002). Negotiating the swamp: The opportunity and challenge of reflexivity in research practice. *Qualitative Research*, 2(2), 209–230. https://doi.org/10.1177/146879410200200205

Fox, M. (2015). Embodied methodologies, participation, and the art of research. *Social and Personality Psychology Compass*, 9(7), 321–332. https://doi.org/10.1111/SPC3.12182

Fricker, M. (2007). *Epistemic injustice: Power and the ethics of knowing*. Oxford University Press.

Graf-Taylor, R. (2012). Philosophy of dialogue and feminist psychology. In M. Friedman (Ed.), *Martin Buber and the human sciences*. State University of New York Press.

Haraway, D. (1988). Situated knowledges: The science question in feminism and the privilege of partial perspective. *Feminist Studies*, 14(3), 575. https://doi.org/10.2307/3178066

Haraway, D. J. (2016). *Staying with the trouble. Making kin in the Chthulucene*. Duke University Press.

Hermans, H. J. M. (2001). The dialogical self: Toward a theory of personal and cultural positioning. *Culture & Psychology*, 7(3), 243–281. https://doi.org/10.1177/1354067X0173001

Hermans, H. J. M. (2022). *Liberation in the face of uncertainty. A new development in dialogical self theory*. Cambridge University Press.

LaMarre, A. (2021). Embodying artistic reflexive praxis: An early career academic's reflections on pain, anxiety, and eating disorder recovery research. *Forum Qualitative Sozialforschung/Forum: Qualitative Social Research*, 22(2). https://doi.org/10.17169/FQS-22.2.3712

Launeanu, M., & Kwee, J. L. (2018). A non-dualistic and existential perspective on understanding and treating disordered eating. In H. L. McBride & J. L. Kwee (Eds.), *Embodiment and eating disorders: Theory, research, prevention, and treatment* (pp. 35–52). Routledge.

Lazard, L., & McAvoy, J. (2020). Doing reflexivity in psychological research: What's the point? What's the practice? *Qualitative Research in Psychology*, 17(2), 159–177. https://doi.org/10.1080/14780887.2017.1400144

Lenz Taguchi, H. (2012). A diffractive and Deleuzian approach to analysing interview data. *Feminist Theory*, 13(3), 265–281. https://doi.org/10.1177/1464700112456001

Mauthner, N. S., & Doucet, A. (2003). Reflexive accounts and accounts of reflexivity in qualitative data analysis. *Sociology*, 37(3), 413–431. https://doi.org/10.1177/00380385030373002

McBride, H. L. (2021). *The wisdom of your body. Finding healing, wholeness, and connection through embodied living*. Baker Publishing Group.

Phoenix, A., & Pattynama, P. (2006). Intersectionality. *European Journal of Women's Studies*, 13(3), 187–192. https://doi.org/10.1177/1350506806065751

Schuman, J., & Galvez, M. (1996). A Meta/Multi-Discursive Reading of 'False Memory Syndrome'. *Feminism & Psychology*, 6(1), 7–29. https://doi.org/10.1177/0959353596061002

Singleton, P. (2020). Remodelling barbie, making justice: An autoethnography of craftivist encounters. *Feminism and Psychology*. https://doi.org/10.1177/0959353520941355

Wilkinson, S. (1988). The role of reflexivity in feminist psychology. *Women's Studies International Forum*, 11(5), 493–502. https://doi.org/10.1016/0277-5395(88)90024-6.

Wilson, S. (2018). Haunting and the knowing and showing of qualitative research. *The Sociological Review*, 66(6), 1209–1225. https://doi.org/10.1177/0038026118769843

9
STAYING WITH AND LOOKING AHEAD

Perhaps
there is deep learning
and unlearning
the kind that happens in stillness
the kind that asks us to stop
for a moment.
Take it all in
process.
put the tools down.
stop.
I am not ready.
And maybe
I am.
'stillness' by Tanya Frances

Introduction

This final chapter provides a critical and reflective overview of the key themes explored in this book. As I write it, I think about how this project began: grappling with difficult realities and turning to theory to make sense of experiences of violence that are deeply woven into personal memory and entangled with socio-political systems and concerns.

> Feminism itself can be understood as an affective inheritance; how our own struggles to make sense of realities that are difficult to grasp become part of a wider struggle, a struggle to be, to make sense of being
> *Ahmed (2017, p. 3)*

This book has considered that, in narrating change and recoveries after childhood domestic violence, multiple influences may not only intersect in young women's lives but can also be irreconcilable. This has implications for understanding young women's developmental trajectories after childhood domestic violence. Through using a dialogical narrative approach, I consider what it means to 'stay with' knowledge-generation practices and processes that are not neat and not linear, and that have the potential to bring about sites of tension and discomfort for storytellers, readers and listeners. I consider the methodological and epistemological impacts of *how* we listen to accounts of domestic violence in childhood, and I think ahead by offering some considerations for listening practices and understanding childhood domestic abuse for researchers, practitioners and policymakers.

Reflecting on epistemic (in)justice

In Chapter 3, I defined epistemic injustice, and I have made links between types of epistemic injustice and women's storytelling practices throughout the book. I want to come back to what epistemic injustice means for a moment, before reflecting on implications for working towards epistemic justice. Epistemic injustice refers to the harm done to a person when their capacity as an epistemic subject (a knower, a reasoner, a questioner or an interpreter) is undermined, and a listener/hearer does not take their knowledge as seriously as they should. Miranda Fricker (2007) proposes that epistemic justice can happen in two ways. She describes testimonial injustice as an issue of identity prejudice and social injustice. It is where a listener's prejudice causes them to afford less credibility to the speaker based on their assumptions and biases relating to the speaker's identity and, thus, the credibility of their accounts. She also proposed that hermeneutical injustice is another kind of epistemic injustice where there is a gap in sense-making resources between a speaker and listener or between social groups. It is where a person may be unable to fully make sense of their own experience, let alone make it communicable and comprehensible to another. Both forms of epistemic injustice are understood as located in broader systems of power, privilege and oppression.

This book has explored how young women I interviewed narrated recoveries and transitions and made sense of their experiences of childhood domestic violence. The women I interviewed had not accessed formal sources of support to address their experiences of domestic violence, even though some spoke about various ways they had tried to seek support or had hoped for their distress to be seen and recognised by adults such as teachers, police or social workers. The fact that women I interviewed had not accessed domestic abuse services or received formal support in this way means that their childhood experiences took place out of the gaze of services or institutions, which might have validated and legitimised their experiences and might have meant that sense-making resources could have been more socially available and shared. In other words, hermeneutical injustice shaped their childhoods. It provided a historical canvas already painted with experiences of being unable to fully comprehend their own experiences or make them communicable or intelligible for others. This hermeneutical injustice can be understood as gendered and age-based. It is situated within socio-cultural contexts that privilege masculine 'adult' knowledge and do not always take the voices of women or children seriously due to assumptions that women may be too unstable or emotional and children are not yet adults, and so lack rationality and maturity. As such, for some women, there were limited ways of talking about the complexities of their experiences of domestic abuse or even naming the violence they experienced as domestic violence or abuse.

Previous research has explored the power of an authorised account of domestic violence, suggesting that professionalised or therapeutic discourses can shape childhood accounts, as these accounts are readable and accepted versions of the violence that happened (Callaghan et al., 2017). These authorised accounts do not always fit with experiences of abuse, and they serve to smoothen out the multivocality of the expression of their experiences. However, authorised accounts also have the capacity to provide stable stories that are more likely to be considered reliable by those who are listening.

Terminology, language and talk about trauma have been popularised in social and cultural discourse through survivor movements such as #MeToo and the increase of efforts to be trauma-informed across communities and health and social care settings (Alcoff, 2018; Elliott et al., 2005; Walkley & Cox, 2013; Zaleski et al., 2016). The popularisation of the language and understanding of trauma means that some might feel able to speak out more about violence that may previously have been considered less speakable. The mainstreaming of talking about trauma also does something to strengthen the survivor discourse that shaped recovery stories. However, it also limits what can be said about surviving violence and it also limits how these stories can be voiced. This speaks to the way that theory-based knowledge is privileged when people speak about the violence they have experienced (Alcoff & Gray, 1993). In various ways, women storied themselves as gaining resilience and strength from their experiences, positioning them in a survivor position, despite the ways that their experiences, in part, transgressed dominant survivor narrative frameworks due to ambivalences, ongoing struggle, emotion that feels 'too much' or still not fully comprehending or making sense of the incomprehensible. This highlights that those whose stories largely exist out of the gaze of institutions, services or digress dominant narrative frameworks are left in an epistemic gap where their experiential knowledge is not counted and has limited ways of being told. Or where the sense-making resources are lacking, and so there are limited ways of understanding the self and making that understanding intelligible to others.

Narrating, resisting and re-inscribing neoliberal and gendered recovery narratives

Neoliberalism refers to an ideology and culture that emphasises individual responsibility and values self-driven 'success' (Ahmed, 2014; Rose, 1992). A critical exploration of neoliberal ideologies helps to recognise the social and political contexts that emphasise individual responsibility, thus making invisible socio-political structures and removing the responsibility of the state to address those (Edwards, 2002). Understanding this work as located within neoliberal times is an acknowledgement that domestic abuse happens within broader social structures that promote individualising frameworks to make sense of domestic abuse, psychological distress and recovery. These single-story narrative frameworks around individual success offer little space for attending to the social, political and relational contexts that also shape how people make sense of, experience and retell experiences of violence.

In various ways, women's accounts were shaped by self-reliance, self-evaluation and a focus on finding inner strength to 'move on', 'forgive and forget' or to become 'stronger' and 'wiser' or 'choose the better life'. In some ways, these stories can be useful to women in offering a sense of empowerment. At the same time, these kinds of recovery stories also re-inscribe neoliberal individualising understandings of 'successful' recovery as an individual endeavour consisting of self-improvement, which only the self is responsible for. This intersects with gendered ideologies of femininity, which already locate womanhood within individualising discourses of self-work and self-improvement (McRobbie, 2004). These are culturally valuable stories to tell, particularly in the aftermath of violence (Alcoff & Gray, 1993). These narrative resources of self-improvement and self-driven success can be useful and help women move through, survive and construct a sense of self that has the capacity to change and the power to do so. Telling a neoliberal recovery story can provide a quality of coherency that has the capacity to stabilise the therapeutic recovered self. However, these individualising narrative frameworks are limiting. They risk women narrating stories in which they alone are responsible for their happiness and recovery, erasing the social, relational and political ways in which recovery and violence are located (Rose, 2010; Wastell & White, 2012). As well as this, individualising psychotherapeutic narrative frameworks can invite all adulthood difficulties to be correlated with the abuse experienced in childhood, and this can limit the diverse voices that constitute recovery stories and how such stories can be articulated and heard.

Young women's childhoods were not simply left behind, and childhood could not easily be narrated as separate from adulthood. Women's stories consisted of entanglements of childhood and adulthood. For example, women's accounts highlighted a lack of a 'guide' or 'blueprint' for how to do adulthood. The way that adulthood difficulties are storied as individual problems that are explained by the 'damage' of the past invites women to write themselves into stories shaped by deficit and damage with limited ways to story a 'better life' in ways that are communicable and intelligible to others.

Stories of getting by, moving on and surviving were messy, sometimes hard to articulate, and sometimes incomprehensible even to the women I spoke with. For example, women's positions as having moved on were central to articulating a story of strength and resilience, but that positioning left little space to express the uncertainties and conflicts many still held. As such, recovery stories were relational and situated, meaning that when we tell our stories and when we listen to the stories of others, these are not neutral spaces. Stories of how we survive and live through violence are told in socio-political contexts, which value a particular kind of recovery story that is linear, stable and has a fixed endpoint of strength and survivorship (Alcoff, 2018). As such, dominant narratives of 'moving on' and being 'stronger and wiser', although useful in some ways, leave little room for conflict, struggle or tension without unsettling the linearity and stability of the story. Attending to polyvocality meant staying with and examining stories that consisted of strength and survivorship and that were simultaneously entangled with stories of struggle and doubt.

Staying with ambiguous, irreconcilable assemblages of voices

Assemblages of voices refers to the multiple co-existing voices that women speak from when narrating childhood domestic violence and processes of change and transition through young adulthood. Remembering, storying and listening to experiences of childhood domestic violence is a dynamic, relational and socio-culturally situated process. 'Staying with' describes what happens when listeners stay with messiness, middle-ness, ambiguity, irreconcilability, tensions and contradictions. I consider that staying with discomfort or such ambiguity and multivocality can also invite us, as listeners, to attend to all forms of knowledge by using bodymind reflexive listening practices.

In navigating young adulthood, change and transition can be understood as dialogical, negotiated and uncertain processes in which the 'I' is not always stable. Drawing on selfhood as dialogical (Hermans, 2001), the concept of 'innovation' suggests the self is unfinalisable, always having the capacity to change and renew. New identity positions such as 'mother', 'adult' or 'partner' can be viewed through a dialogical lens of innovation. Drawing on Zittoun's (2007) theorisation of transitions as fluid, unfinalisable and ongoing processes of identity work and development, shaped by socio-culturally available symbolic resources, these identity positions can provide access to new cultural resources, and they can present opportunities to re-story the self into resistance and hope for change. For example, the perceived deficits of women's own childhoods could be re-storied as having the potential to offer opportunities for change. From a new mother identity, women such as Bethany could re-construct the self as emotionally distanced from their childhood. A re-construction like this can be useful in providing a distance that took her away from the instability and violence of her childhood, and it offers a sense of narrative agency about how her future mothering might be. Oberman and Josselson (1996) proposed that becoming a mother is a series of dialectical tensions – they theorise a matrix of tensions, one of which speaks to these findings: simultaneous loss of self and sense of expansion. This loss of self, or distance from a childhood self, also exists alongside potential expansion and innovation, enabling the possibility that childhood violence does not have to lead to adulthood instability.

The dialogical approach I used in this work offered useful and generative opportunities. It offered a way of challenging binary distinctions, such as struggle and strength or agency and fragility. I found that working with the Listening Guide and making and working with voice poems helped explore more overt and hidden voices while problematising binary constructions of voice (Harel-Shalev & Daphna-Tekoah, 2021). 'Staying with' the co-existence of overt and more marginalised voices can be a valuable and generative practice for knowledge production. Feminist scholars have argued that we need to adopt feminist listening and analytic practices that support women's meaning-making and narrative practices. Especially, if there is a risk that particular voices will become marginalised or silenced. In listening to accounts of childhood domestic violence, we can learn from feminist listening practices by engaging with and learning from nuances, listening beyond words and dwelling in the silences and places where words can fail women (Chadwick, 2017; Mauthner, 2017; McKenzie-Mohr & Lafrance, 2011; Woodcock, 2016).

When listening to and making sense of women's narratives of childhood domestic violence and transitions to young adulthood, staying with the 'I' meant continuously tracing multiple voices as they threaded through women's accounts. Drawing on the assumption that the personal and political are entangled and interrelated in the practice and process of storytelling, a dialogical and creative approach to working with women's narratives supported the resistance of an individualising philosophy of the self. Attending to the polyvocality of women's stories became an important methodological and ontological practice. This practice enabled me to reject a single unitary self-logic. Rather than assuming that 'I' is stable, authentic and singular, I worked with the idea of the self as multiple, fluid and expressed polyvocally

(Sermijn et al., 2008). Through this way of working with stories, I found I could find ways 'in' to stay with voices that I may not have ordinarily heard or tuned into. Through this listening practice, I have explored that recovery stories were not fixed, and they consisted of nuances and marginalised voices such as shame, doubt, uncertainty, loss and hope. However, articulating these nuances risks producing incoherence in the narrative, destabilising the recovery story, and producing an unstable 'I'.

Thinking ahead: considerations for research, policy and practice

Before offering concluding thoughts, I consider how this book might speak to researchers, practitioners and policymakers. However, firstly, I want to highlight the limitations of the book. The research I conducted has limitations as specific demographic information was not formally gathered from participants, such as sexual orientation, faith, ethnicity and disability. It is likely that a more attuned intersectional analytic would have been possible if more detailed demographic information had been gathered. This is much needed in domestic violence research. While information was disclosed and discussed in interviews, this was as-and-when it came up as part of the interview rather than formally gathered. Therefore, the analysis is only attuned to identities that were voiced during interviews. I join others in calling for analytics that take up an intersectional lens, with more diverse sample in research about childhood domestic violence (Etherington & Baker, 2018).

My interest in the impact of narrating childhood domestic abuse and transitions to young adulthood, particularly in neoliberal times, serves to turn attention to the interrelatedness of psychology and politics in the context of recovery after childhood violence, distress and trauma (Moncrieff et al., 2011). Children and families who experience adversities, including domestic violence, are still predominantly positioned in problematic ways in social, clinical and academic discourses (see an overview in Överlien & Holt, 2018). Experiencing domestic violence is impactful and traumatic in many ways that extend far beyond words. However, a single-story viewpoint is rarely helpful, particularly when it provides a narrative framework shaped by deficit and damage and offers little space for alternative stories to be voiced.

This book has taken seriously that, often, when women talk about experiences of violence or abuse, their accounts risk being smoothened or flattened out to a single storyline, neglecting the multiplicity of their stories and identities. Domestic abuse is an issue that people might seek formal support or justice for in a variety of ways and contexts, for instance, in health and social care, education, criminal justice or legal systems, specialist domestic or sexual violence services or counselling and psychological services (Holt et al.,

2017; Howarth et al., 2015; Lombard & McMillan, 2013). In all these contexts, particularly in criminal justice and legal systems, it is well known that survivors face barriers to being heard, believed and listened to as credible self-narrators, with huge implications for their mental health, including high rates of retraumatisation (Herman, 2003). Moreover, women and children from already marginalised backgrounds and identities face additional barriers when seeking safety or justice (Action for Children, 2019; Austin, 2021).

Compounding these issues is that incident or act-based conceptualisations and understandings of domestic abuse within legal and criminal justice systems serve to invisibilise the gendered and patriarchal structures that characterise and underpin domestic abuse (Burman & Brooks-Hay, 2018; Stark & Hester, 2019). I highlight these issues to show the importance of attending to epistemic injustices in domestic violence research, practice and policymaking. To avoid reproducing oppression and marginalisation through the methods and listening practices we use, it is crucial that research with survivors centres a diverse range of voices. It is crucial that we do not use methods that only make space for hearing what is most communicable, comprehensible and intelligible and that we intentionally embrace listening practices that offer opportunities to 'stay with' discomfort, ambiguities, hesitancies and explore them.

My hope is that domestic abuse policies, legislation and practices work to recognise and account for the socio-structural conditions that enable violence and, importantly, the social, structural and relational conditions that can help people recover and make meaning out of their experiences in useful ways. In thinking ahead, I invite researchers and practitioners to consider how they work with and attend to ambiguities and tensions and how they listen to and work with human experience that is multiple and polyvocal. In previous writing, I have considered particular implications for counsellors and psychotherapists (Frances, 2024). These practical implications extend to clinicians and legal professionals who work with those who experience childhood domestic violence in terms of attending to the risk of pathologising women's uncertainties and buying into and re-inscribing dominant and gendered discourses about adulthood, survival and growing up after childhood domestic violence. I also join calls for more support to be available to those who experience childhood domestic violence and for practitioners to work with how experiences of domestic violence shape gendered and intersectional identities into adulthood (Levell, 2022).

Concluding thoughts

In the spirit of dialogical thinking, I find myself thinking about unfinalisability. This work is ongoing, and as such, I welcome the fact that it is not easy to summarise conclusions in a neat and absolute way. To assist with offering concluding thoughts, I return to Sara Ahmed's thinking about living out feminism:

> feminism brings to mind loud acts of refusal and rebellion as well as the quiet ways we might have of not holding onto things that diminish us.
> *(Ahmed, 2017, p. 1)*

This reckoning with feminism and definition of feminism resonates with me and perhaps says something about how we tune into both the loud and quiet ways that women give voice to who we are in the aftermath of violence. Re-storying the self after domestic violence in childhood can be a tentative and uncertain process and practice, particularly when stories resist dominant 'expert' discourses that carry epistemological power. This book has explored the interplay of dialogical voices within young women's narratives, suggesting that not only can conflict, tension and ambiguity within storied accounts be important sites of knowledge, but they can also present irreconcilable tensions. Narrating both struggle and 'success' can, at times, become a narrative impossibility. Polyvocal narratives about change and transition in young adulthood after childhood domestic violence both re-inscribe societal narratives of insecurity and doubt as well as present stories of resistance and hope. Transition and change stories can be powerful, hopeful and mobilising as well as simultaneously, limiting and constraining. Rather than construct this instability and unfinalisability as pathology, or a sign of deficit, narrative instability can be considered an important site of knowledge.

The human capacity to change and to re-story the self over time can be expressed in diverse, loud and quiet ways. Assuming that the psychological and political are entangled and interrelated in the practice and process of storytelling, a dialogical approach offers opportunities to resist an individualising philosophy of the self, and it can offer an alternative way of making sense of young women's experiences through and after domestic violence in childhood.

This book aligns with feminist scholars who have argued for the importance of attending to multiplicity (Chadwick, 2020; Mauthner, 2017), marginalised voices and epistemological injustices (Fine, 2012) and examining the socio-cultural conditions and resources that shape how women voice accounts of violence (Gavey, 2018; Hydén, 2005; Nicolson, 2019). This book contributes to existing qualitative literature about childhood domestic violence by offering a critical feminist psychological perspective that examines gendered and socio-culturally located storytelling practices. While this is a very well-argued position by feminist violence researchers, this book calls for more researchers to take a critical analytical lens to examine socio-culturally located dynamics of power when understanding childhood domestic violence. It also calls for considerations of recovery after violence that account for context, community, collectiveness, creativity and multiplicity.

References

Action for Children. (2019). *Patchy, piecemeal and precarious: Support for children affected by domestic abuse*. https://media.actionforchildren.org.uk/documents/patchy-piecemeal-and-precarious-support-for-children-affected-by-domestic-abuse.pdf

Ahmed, S. (2014). *The cultural politics of emotion* (2nd ed.). Edinburgh University Press.

Ahmed, S. (2017). *Living a feminist life*. Duke University Press.

Alcoff, L. (2018). *Rape and resistance*. Polity Press.

Alcoff, L., & Gray, L. (1993). Survivor discourse: Transgression or recuperation? *Signs: Journal of Women in Culture and Society, 18*(2), 260–290. https://doi.org/10.1086/494793

Austin, J. (2021). *Nowhere to turn 2021 report*. https://www.womensaid.org.uk/womens-aid-launches-nowhere-to-turn-2021-report-findings-from-the-fifth-year-of-the-no-woman-turned-away-project/

Burman, M., & Brooks-Hay, O. (2018). Aligning policy and law? The creation of a domestic abuse offence incorporating coercive control. *Criminology & Criminal Justice, 18*(1), 67–83. https://doi.org/10.1177/1748895817752223

Callaghan, J. E. M., Fellin, L. C., Mavrou, S., Alexander, J., & Sixsmith, J. (2017). The management of disclosure in children's accounts of domestic violence: Practices of telling and not telling. *Journal of Child and Family Studies, 26*(12), 3370–3387. https://doi.org/10.1007/s10826-017-0832-3

Chadwick, R. (2017). Embodied methodologies: Challenges, reflections and strategies. *Qualitative Research, 17*(1), 54–74. https://doi.org/10.1177/1468794116656035

Chadwick, R. (2020). Methodologies of voice: Towards posthuman voice analytics. *Methods in Psychology, 2*. https://doi.org/10.1016/j.metip.2020.100021

Edwards, R. (2002). *Children, home, and school regulation, autonomy or connection?* Routledge.

Elliott, D. E., Bjelajac, P., Fallot, R. D., Markoff, L. S., & Reed, B. G. (2005). Trauma-informed or trauma-denied: Principles and implementation of trauma-informed services for women. *Journal of Community Psychology, 33*(4), 461–477. https://doi.org/10.1002/jcop.20063

Etherington, N., & Baker, L. (2018). From "buzzword" to best practice: Applying intersectionality to children exposed to intimate partner violence. *Trauma, Violence, & Abuse, 19*(1), 58–75. https://doi.org/10.1177/1524838016631128

Fine, M. (2012). Troubling calls for evidence: A critical race, class and gender analysis of whose evidence counts. *Feminism & Psychology, 22*(1), 3–19. https://doi.org/10.1177/0959353511435475

Frances, T. (2024). A dialogical narrative approach to transitions and change in young women's lives after domestic abuse in childhood: Considerations for counselling and psychotherapy. *British Journal of Guidance & Counselling, 52*(1), 19–35.

Fricker, M. (2007). *Epistemic injustice: Power and the ethics of knowing*. Oxford University Press.

Gavey, N. (2018). *Just sex?: The cultural scaffolding of rape* (2nd ed.). Routledge.

Harel-Shalev, A., & Daphna-Tekoah, S. (2021). Breaking the binaries in research - the listening guide. *Qualitative Psychology, 8*(2), 211–223. https://doi.org/10.1037/QUP0000201

Herman, J. L. (2003). The mental health of crime victims: Impact of legal intervention. *Journal of Traumatic Stress*, 16(2), 159–166. https://doi.org/10.1023/A:1022847223135

Hermans, H. J. M. (2001). The dialogical self: Toward a theory of personal and cultural positioning. *Culture & Psychology*, 7(3), 243–281. https://doi.org/10.1177/1354067X0173001

Holt, S., Overlien, C., & Devaney, J. (2017). *Responding to domestic violence. Emerging challenges for policy, practice and research in Europe*. Jessica Kingsley Publishers.

Howarth, E., Moore, T. H. M., Shaw, A. R. G., Welton, N. J., Feder, G. S., Hester, M., MacMillan, H. L., & Stanley, N. (2015). The effectiveness of targeted interventions for children exposed to domestic violence: Measuring success in ways that matter to children, parents and professionals. *Child Abuse Review*, 24(4), 297–310. https://doi.org/10.1002/car.2408

Hydén, M. (2005). 'I must have been an idiot to let it go on': Agency and positioning in battered women's narratives of leaving. *Feminism & Psychology*, 15(2), 169–188. https://doi.org/10.1177/0959353505051725

Levell, J. (2022). *Boys, childhood, domestic abuse and gang involvement*. Bristol University Press.

Lombard, N., & McMillan, L. (2013). *Violence against women. Current theory and practice in domestic abuse, sexual violence, and exploitation*. Jessica Kingsley Publishers.

Mauthner, N. S. (2017). The listening guide feminist method of narrative analysis: Towards a posthumanist performative (re)configuration. In J. Woodiwiss, K. Smith, & K. Lockwood (Eds.), *Feminist narrative research: Opportunities and challenges* (pp. 65–91). Palgrave Macmillan UK.

McKenzie-Mohr, S., & Lafrance, M. N. (2011). Telling stories without the words: 'Tightrope talk' in women's accounts of coming to live well after rape or depression. *Feminism & Psychology*, 21(1), 49–73. https://doi.org/10.1177/0959353510371367

McRobbie, A. (2004). Post-feminism and popular culture. *Feminist Media Studies*, 4(3), 255–264. https://doi.org/10.1080/1468077042000309937

Moncrieff, J., Rapley, M., & Dillon, J. (2011). *De-medicalizing misery: Psychiatry, psychology and the human condition*. Palgrave Macmillan.

Nicolson, P. (2019). *Domestic violence and psychology: Critical perspectives on intimate partner violence and abuse*. Routledge.

Oberman, Y., & Josselson, R. (1996). Matrix of tensions: A model of mothering. *Psychology of Women Quarterly*, 20(3), 341–359. https://doi.org/10.1111/J.1471-6402.1996.TB00304.X

Överlien, C., & Holt, S. (2018). Letter to the editor: Research on children experiencing domestic violence. *Journal of Family Violence*, 34(1), 65–67. https://doi.org/10.1007/s10896-018-9997-9

Rose, N. (1992). "Governing the enterprising self." In P. Heelas & P. Morris (Eds.), *The values of the enterprise culture: The moral debate* (pp. 141–164). Routledge.

Rose, N. (2010). 'Screen and intervene': Governing risky brains. *History of the Human Sciences*, 23(1), 79–105. https://doi.org/10.1177/0952695109352415

Sermijn, J., Devlieger, P., & Loots, G. (2008). The narrative construction of the self. *Qualitative Inquiry*, 14(4), 632–650. https://doi.org/10.1177/1077800408314356

Stark, E., & Hester, M. (2019). Coercive control: Update and review. *Violence Against Women, 25*(1), 81–104. https://doi.org/10.1177/1077801218816191

Walkley, M., & Cox, T. L. (2013). Building trauma-informed schools and communities. *Children & Schools, 35*(2), 123–126. https://doi.org/10.1093/cs/cdt007

Wastell, D., & White, S. (2012). Blinded by neuroscience: Social policy, the family and the infant brain. *Families, Relationships and Societies, 1*(3), 397–414. https://doi.org/10.1332/204674312X656301

Woodcock, C. (2016). The listening guide. *International Journal of Qualitative Methods, 15*(1), 1–10. https://doi.org/10.1177/1609406916677594

Zaleski, K. L., Johnson, D. K., & Klein, J. T. (2016). Grounding Judith Herman's trauma theory within interpersonal neuroscience and evidence-based practice modalities for trauma treatment. *Smith College Studies in Social Work, 86*(4), 377–393. https://doi.org/10.1080/00377317.2016.1222110

Zittoun, T. (2007). Symbolic resources and responsibility in transitions. *Young, 15*(2), 193–211. https://doi.org/10.1177/110330880701500205

INDEX

Note: Page numbers followed by "n" denote endnotes.

Action for Children 5
adulthood: after domestic violence 11–13; autonomy 72, 76; health-risk behaviour in 15; instability 64, 142; rationality 72; resilience and wellness in 18
'adverse childhood experience' (ACE) 15–17, 22n1
age-based markers 77
Ahmed, S. 34–35, 93, 119, 137, 145
ambiguous/irreconcilable assemblages of voices 141–143
Anderson, K. M. 12
anti-feminist 30
assemblages: ambiguous/irreconcilable 141–143; of voices 141–143
attention deficit hyperactivity disorder (ADHD) assessment 83–85
authenticity: quest for 85–91; and self-work 85–91
authentic voice 53–54, 126, 133

Bakhtin, M. 51
'better life' 81, 91–94, 97, 105, 128, 140, 141
blueprints 66–69, 78, 141
bodymind listening 123–124

Cambridge Dictionary 101
Carrick, D. 2

Chadwick, R. 113, 132
change: domestic violence 20–21; socio-cultural perspective 20–21; and transitions 20–21
childhood: after domestic violence 11–13; domestic violence in 3–6; as not simply 'witnesses' to violence 10–11
conflict 96, 100, 110, 118–119, 141, 145
Couzens, W. 2
Crime Survey for England and Wales (CSEW) data 2, 4

Danis, F. S. 12
de-centralisation of self-knowledge 53
deficit model of development 14
dialogical listeners 125–126
dialogical philosophy 55, 125
dialogical relationships 64, 72, 76, 93, 126
dialogical self 51, 52, 64
Dialogical Self Theory 8, 51, 52, 66, 72, 74, 77, 91, 125, 126
domestic abuse 2–7, 10, 11, 14, 15, 19, 43–45, 54, 81, 89, 91, 138–140, 143, 144
Domestic Abuse Act (2021) 4–5, 11
domestic violence 3–4, 16, 97; 'adverse childhood experience' 15–17; change and transitions 20–21; in childhood 3–6; from childhood to

adulthood 11–13; children as not simply 'witnesses' to violence 10–11; resilience 13–15; resilient brains/resilient people 17–20; socio-cultural perspective 20–21
domestic violence and abuse (DVA) 3, 13, 37
dominant narrative resources 61, 65, 103, 104, 117
Dumont, A. 13, 22
dysfunction 15, 22n1, 67–68
dysfunctional relationships 67–68

Edleson, J. L. 6
embodied knowledge 132–134
embodied listening 122–135
embodiment 17, 37, 122, 124
empiricism 32
epistemic injustice 31–34; defined 138; reflecting on 138–140
epistemic justice 3, 7, 8, 22, 31, 33, 122–135, 138; bodymind listening as work toward 123–124; defined 33; embodied knowledge 132–134; listeners as dialogical and always-changing selves 125–126; listening as slow process 126–128; relational knowledge 132–134; staying with stuckness 128–132
Everard, S. 2

False Memory Syndrome 29–31, 37
Felitti, A. 15, 16
feminism 28, 31, 50, 145; as a life question 34–37; Western 34
feminist: dialogical approach 41, 50–54, 57; informed therapists 30; listening 54, 142; psychologists 19, 34–35; psychology 3, 7, 22, 30
forgetting 94–96
forgiving 94–96
Fox, M. 133
Frank, A. 42, 50, 56
Fricker, M. 33, 122, 138

gender: -based inequalities 19; feminist psychological perspective on 28–38; importance of 28–31; socio-structural forces 117
gendered recovery narratives: narrating 140–141; re-inscribing 140–141; resisting 140–141
Global North 1, 6, 7

Gonzales, G. 12
Graham-Bermann, S. A. 6
The Guardian 1

Haraway, D. 36, 134
Hermans, H. 51–53
hermeneutical injustice 3, 33, 110, 111, 117, 118, 126, 138–139
historical legacies 28–31
hope: tentative 66–69; as voice of resistance 68
Humphreys, C. 11
Hydén, M. 96

identity 3, 13, 19, 21, 33, 34, 45, 48, 52–53, 56, 64, 77, 85, 88, 91, 96, 138
independent lives 51, 64
injustice: epistemic 31–34, 138–140; hermeneutical 3, 33, 110, 111, 117, 118, 126, 138–139; social 33, 36, 138; testimonial 3, 33, 93, 122, 128, 130–131, 134, 138
innovation 53–54, 56, 142
innovation of self 53–54
interviewer–interviewee relationship 124
interviews 45–49

Jefferson, A. M. 32
Josselson, R. 64, 142
justice: epistemic 122–135; social 133

knowledge: embodied 132–134; objective 32, 36; relational 132–134; scientific 22; self-knowledge 53; subjective 32

Lafrance, M. N. 103, 112
Lessard, G. 13, 22
Levell, J. 13, 16, 22
listeners: as always-changing selves 125–126; as dialogical 125–126
listening: bodymind 123–124; embodied 122–135; reflexive 122–135; as slow process 126–128
Listening Guide 54–56, 123, 142

Macleod, C. 34
marginalised voices 6, 42, 118, 133, 135, 142, 145
McKenzie-Mohr, S. 103, 112
memory 28–31; 'False Memory Syndrome' 29–31, 37; feminist

psychological perspective on 28–38; personal 137; recall 29; 'recovered' 30
'memory wars' 37
mental illness 19, 81, 82, 89
metaphors 101–104, 119
#MeToo 1, 139
mother–child relationships 10, 19
motherhood 107; transitions to 62–66
mothering 63, 64, 78, 116
Motzkau, J. F. 32
Moulding, N. T. 117
Mullender, A. 6
multiplicity: of meanings 41; in unity 53–54, 74
multivocality/polyvocality 37, 49–50, 97, 134–135, 139, 141
Musk, E. 42
myth of objectivity 22, 32

narrating survival: as a battle 105–107; when there is potential to be misunderstood 112–114
narrative 41–42; gendered recovery narratives 140–141; neoliberal recovery narratives 140–141; psychology 100; strategies 6, 8, 100, 101, 118; 'thinking narratively' 49–50
National Police Chief's Council (NPCC) 1–2
National Society for the Prevention of Cruelty to Children (NSPCC) 4–5
neoliberalism 140
neoliberal recovery narratives: narrating 140–141; re-inscribing 140–141; resisting 140–141
Nicholson, P. 37
non-violent relationship 14

Oberman, Y. 61, 142
objective knowledge 32, 36
objective 'scientific' evidence 133
O'Brien, K. L. 12
ontological (in)security 107–111

patriarchal structures 2, 37, 131, 144
Peled, E. 6
poems: creating 54–56; Listening Guide 54–56; voice 54–56; working with 54–56
power: cultural 73, 103; economic 19, 34; epistemic 101; epistemological 22, 66, 145; institutional 19, 34; political 19, 34, 103; and recovery stories 97–98; relations 2, 32, 35–36, 42, 50; re-negotiations of 73–77; social 18, 72–73, 103; structures 6
precarious work 100–120; chess and black holes 101–104; and creative assemblages of voice/s 100–120; narrating survival 105–107, 112–114; ontological (in)security 107–111; sense-making 114–118; storying tensions/contradictions through metaphor 101–104
psychotherapeutic narrative resource 80–84

recovery narratives: gendered 140–141; neoliberal 140–141
recovery/recoveries 80–98; forgiving/ forgetting/moving on 94–96; and power 97–98; resilience and choosing 'better life' 91–94; self-work and authenticity 85–91; storying self as psychotherapeutic subject 81–85
reflexive listening 122–135
reflexivity 57, 122, 124–125, 131, 134, 135
re-inscribing: gendered recovery narratives 140–141; neoliberal recovery narratives 140–141
relational 13; approach 123; beings 134; contexts 18, 29, 57, 76, 125, 140; dynamics 4, 66; and embodied forms of knowledge 132–134; method 54; philosophy 134; process 19, 29, 141; and socio-cultural 3; space 48; theory of transitions/change 61, 77; way of listening 55
relational knowledge 132–134
relationships: dialogical 64, 72, 76, 93, 126; dysfunctional 67–68; interviewer–interviewee relationship 124; long-term 67; mother–child relationship 10, 19; non-violent relationship 14; supportive 12, 19; traditional 62
resilience 13–15; and choosing the 'better life' 91–94; resilient brains 17–20; resilient people 17–20
resistance 12, 17, 42, 54, 76, 78, 125, 127, 132, 134–135, 145; gendered recovery narratives 140–141; neoliberal recovery narratives 140–141

scientific knowledge 22
self/selves: always-changing 125–126; contradictions 118; evaluative structure 81, 82, 84, 85; innovation of 53–54; integrations 118; knowledge 53, 90, 94; negotiations 118; as psychotherapeutic subject 81–85; work 85–91
selves-in-relation 134
sense-making 114–118
sexual violence 4, 29, 43, 104, 143
Singleton, P. 124
social injustice 33, 36, 138
social justice 133
socially structured human activity 29
socio-cultural relational theory 61, 77
socio-cultural theorisation 21
stories 41–42; self as psychotherapeutic subject 81–85; tensions/contradictions through metaphor 101–104
subjective knowledge 32
substance use problems 19
supportive relationships 12, 19
survival 14, 93–94, 100–101; as a battle 105–107; narrating 105–107, 112–114
Suzuki, S. L. 12
Swift, T. 1

Taguchi, L. 124, 132
tensions 101–104
tentative hope 66–69
testimonial injustice 3, 33, 93, 122, 128, 130–131, 134, 138
'the-other-in-self' 52
'thinking narratively' 49–50
traditional relationships 62
transitions 61–78; blueprints and tentative hope 66–69; and change 20–21; domestic violence 20–21; getting older and expressions of voice 70–73; 'I' as adult and re-negotiations of power 73–77; socio-cultural perspective 20–21; transitions to 62–66
'truth' 31–34
Twitter 42–43

United Nations Convention on the Rights of the Child (UNCRC) 6

VAWG National Policing Statement 1
violence: children as not simply 'witnesses' to 10–11; domestic 3–6; remembering/talking about 31–34; 'truth' and epistemic (in)justice 31–34
Violence Against Women and Girls (VAWG) 1–2
voice poems 8, 77, 122–126, 132–135, 142; creating 54–56; developing typologies 56–57; Listening Guide 54–56; working with 54–56
voice/s: ambiguous, irreconcilable assemblages of 141–143; creative assemblages of 100–120; feminist psychological perspective on 28–38; getting older and expressions of 70–73; and precarious work 100–120

Western feminisms 34
Wilson, S. 128
Women's Aid 2, 4–5
Woodiwiss, J. 32, 84, 87
World Health Organization 4

young adulthood 3, 6, 8, 56, 62, 68–69, 73, 76, 85, 88, 104, 141–143, 145

Zittoun, T. 21, 61, 77, 141

For Product Safety Concerns and Information please contact our EU representative GPSR@taylorandfrancis.com
Taylor & Francis Verlag GmbH, Kaufingerstraße 24, 80331 München, Germany